EASY DETOX

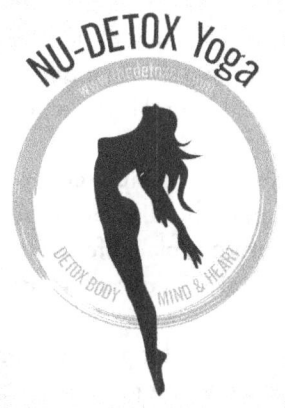

Transform in just 7 days!

DETOX GODDESS 'AT HOME DETOX KIT'
7-DAY DETOX CLEANSE

Printed in the USA, January 2014 ©
ISBN 978-1494376918

1. SHORT INTRODUCTION

Scientists have identified over 72,000 toxins that can pose serious threats to our daily life. Whether it is through the food and water that we ingest, the air that we breathe, or the environment in general, the dangers of over exposure to heavy metals, chemicals and other toxic matters are significant and the imbalances that they create have a measurable negative impact on our energy level, health and overall physical, mental and emotional wellbeing.

In light of our inability to completely neutralize exposure and the alarming increase in life threatening degenerative diseases and conditions more and more people suffer from in our modern societies, the process of detoxification / cleansing has become the only viable solution to limit exposure, reduce the impact of prior exposure, and thereby prevent long term damage to our immune system, individual organs and overall health and longevity. Detox has become a necessary strategy for optimum health & wellness.

So detox is not just a 'fad', and while juicing companies have sprouted everywhere to take full advantage of the increased awareness in educated consumers around the subject of over-toxicity and the consequential ill-health, the process is completely legitimate and useful.

That said, detox is a natural process that is solely performed by the body when it is not overloaded with toxins and when proper nutrition is available for the body to perform its natural detox function. That is what Easy Detox and our Detox Goddess kits were designed for, i.e. to support those processes.

Easy Detox is a step-by-step manual that supports a most enjoyable and practical experience through a proven, simple and highly effective detoxification program, and all of it in the comfort of your own home. And it is perfectly suited to brand new beginners in the field of detox and cleansing too!

In this manual, you'll find instructions to follow a simple detox that fits both your current lifestyle and goals. Having implemented life-changing health and wellness programs in both private and corporate settings for over 12 years now, author and owner at The Detox Co, Alessandrina Lerner knows that to be successful in any venture comes down to how realistic a program is. If it cannot be easily integrated into your current living habits, you will not stick to it. It's that simple! So how can it be done?

Well, all change and personal transformation require an impetus; i.e. the trigger that enables permanent changes to take place - however big or more modest the shift might be. So, what comes next?

Once you've been triggered, you now need to have a feasible program that you'll be able to stick to in the long run, i.e. one that will motivate you to continue to grow both in health and awareness. Once you've had that experience, you now have a point of reference to go back to when making choices.

Ascended spiritual masters such as Jesus and Buddha both emphasized the importance and value of personal experience and inner exploration as a basis for making the 'right' choice.
age
It was Buddha who said, "Believe nothing, no matter where you read it, or who said it, no matter if I have said it, unless it agrees with your own reason and your own common sense."

This book offers 4 flexible detox programs, that you can use with our At Home Detox Kits, or as a stand-alone, that cater to people with different objectives and lifestyles and who have one objective in common; i.e. to Transform their Life through the process of Detoxification.

So whether you chose to detox through a healthier and more balanced diet and approach to healthy living or go all the way with a full on detox juice cleanse, you will gain benefits and you will experience improvement from your current situation and circumstances that will lead you to better and healthier choices day after day,

We hope you enjoy the journey as much as the destination, both are the reason you are here reading this now!

2.   BIO AUTHOR

Alessandrina Lerner is a teacher, consultant, and leader of a team of brilliant professionals who create practical and advanced detox solutions. For over 12 years, she has been been designing wellness programs for both professionals and individuals who seek to improve their health, fitness level and lifestyle. She started her career in holistic health with Swami Brahmavidyananda Saraswati, Director of the Institute for Holistic Yoga, from the lineage of the internationally renowned Indian guru, Swami Sivananda Saraswati who trained her in Hatha Yoga, Breathing Techniques, Meditation and Vegetarian Nutrition. She is also a plant-based and superfoods nutrition counseling consultant, registered as an E-RYT-200 with the Yoga Alliance, a Reiki Level 1 and Reiki Tummo Level 1 & 2 Practitioner, and certified as a provider of TLP, a therapeutic sound/ music stimulation program aimed at restoring auditory functions, enhancing brain functioning, and improving mental and physical well-being. Prior to founding The Detox Co., she co-owned and single-handedly run The South Beach Detox for over 2 years. She lived in a Buddhist temple where she learnt the science of the mind and meditation as a way to transcendence and self-empowerment. She was initiated into Light & Sound Meditation in the tradition of Guru Nanak in 2002 and received empowerment in Tibetan Buddhism (Medicine Buddha and White Tara) in 2012. Her business background is in finance, having held high management positions at American Express, Citicorp/ Citibank and Visa International; with an MBA in International Finance & Strategic Marketing and a BS in Economic & Political Sciences from France leading university, Université Paris IX Dauphine. Experiencing other cultures inspires her, both in her personal and professional life. Her visits to over 60 countries have broadened her perspective of the deeper meaning of existence and have given her the ability to relate to people in ways that she could have never imagined. She shares as much of the knowledge she has gained as she can through her daily work and her writings. So far she has written 7 books, which include two manuals on detoxification, a book on yoga, a novel and three poetry books. She also blogs and tweets regularly about healthy living, enlightenment, and personal empowerment. For more information on Alessandrina Lerner and her detox programs, please visit www.thedetoxco.com. or check The Detox Co's Facebook page at http://tinyurl.com/detoxco.

3. WELCOME NOTE

Welcome to your Detox Goddess 'At Home Detox Kit' and congratulations on your decision to enjoy a balanced and healthy diet and lifestyle.

A detox program is the perfect opportunity to hit the restart button and initiate new beginnings after having cleansed the body of excess toxins, waste material and unwanted debris that might have accumulated in your system throughout your entire life.

Whether you are aware of it or not, this constant strain constitutes a major hindrance to your overall health and wellbeing as the energy that is usually used for optimum functioning of your entire body-mind system is instead being redirected to support the elimination of excessive concentration of pathogens and undesirable debris in the body as well as other stress factors. This continuously drains you of your energy, life-force and vitality and in time adversely impacts your immune system too, leaving you open to illnesses, diseases and mental and emotional imbalances.

Before you begin your detox program, we strongly suggest that you take a few days to prepare for your detox - at least 1, so that you may transition smoothly into the detoxification process. All the necessary information to facilitate this process has been included in the Pre-detox instructions section of this booklet.

To learn more about the detoxification process and the crucial role it plays in keeping you healthy, balanced and content, read the next section 'About Detox' below.

4. TABLE OF CONTENT

5. ABOUT DETOX

What is Detox?

The detoxification process – not just of drugs and alcohol, but of all substances both organic and inorganic that are can be toxic to the body both in high, and sometimes even low levels of concentration (in the case of highly harmful chemicals, metals, etc.), is a natural process whereby the organs (skin, lungs, liver, kidneys, spleen, pancreas, stomach, colon, bladder, etc.) rid themselves of excess toxic build-ups in the body.

What is Toxic Build-Up?

Over time, toxins, waste material, and also negative feelings and emotions that induce physical contraction in the physical body begin to accumulate and create energetic blockages in the different body layers. Without proper release, this greatly affects the normal functioning of various bodily organs and also over taxes the immune system, exposing us to the risk of undesirable conditions developing in the physical, mental and emotional bodies.

While eating a healthy, varied diet and exercising regularly are good stepping stones in the attainment of a desirable level of health and wellbeing, it is seldom enough unless you happen to live in an extremely preserved and uncontaminated part of the world. Modern day living and excessive exposure to stress and toxins through food, water, air and other environmental factors continuously deplete our body, immunity and overtime create havoc in our health whether it be physical, mental or emotional. Under those circumstances, it is becoming increasingly difficult for the body to function optimally, let alone support the natural detoxification process that is necessary to enjoy a healthy and balanced life.

Why Detox?

In light of the excessive toxic exposure that constantly depletes our bodies and minds of the necessary energy they need to function properly, performing regular detox programs or integrating daily detox measures into our daily lives has become a requisite to health and longevity. Having a regular exercise program that emphasizes the detoxification process and maximizes detox benefits is also key to preventing any undue stress to the body and attaining a dynamic and vibrant state of health.

While regular exercise helps promote optimal lymphatic drainage to rid the body of excess toxic waste and deposits, a more in-depth exercise program that also promotes optimal organ functioning and supports natural detoxification is necessary to obtain both measurable and durable results.

The Detox Yoga series and the exclusive Nu-Detox Yoga program were developed with this particular objective in mind. Both programs were designed to support any detox program, so that you may attain optimum detoxification results and maintain optimum health on all levels of your being no matter where you are and when you need it the most.

What is Detox Yoga?

Detox Yoga is a series of 4 instructional yoga classes that are designed to gradually take you deeper into the detoxification process.

The Detox Yoga series incorporates physical postures, breathing exercises, relaxation and meditational techniques – including inner visualization, that are most effective in supporting detoxification on the physical, mental and emotional levels of your being.

Each class builds upon the prior-level class so that you are getting deeper into the detoxification effects and benefits each time through the integration of more advanced variations of basic detox poses, breathing and relaxation exercises and also learning new and more challenging and effective techniques each time.

What is Nu-Detox Yoga?

Nu-Detox Yoga is a creative new branding of yoga, which ingenuously integrates the highly effective disciplines of Qi Gong, Kundalini Yoga, Power Vinyasa, Powerful Breathing techniques, and unique Meditations that are derived from Kriya Yoga, Taoism, Tantrism and Reiki Tummo Healing. The Breathing and Qi Gong portions of this program integrate some of the most powerful practices in Taoism and Qi Gong, as cultivated and refined by Dr. Daniel Atchison-Nevel of www.NSEVhealing.com, and Tao Semko and Santiago Dobles of www.UmaaTantra.com.

6. MAIN DETOX BENEFITS

The benefits most frequently reported by customers who follow one of our private or at home detox programs include;

Physical Benefits
- Increased Energy, Vitality, Endurance and Stamina
- Weight Loss/ L.T. Weight Management (1lb/day - 0.5 kg/day)
- Improved Complexion and Glow
- Improved Bowel Function & Digestion
- Enhanced Immunity and Better Health
- Decreased Stress & Better Sleep
- New Healthy Eating Habits

Mental Benefits
- Increased Focus & Concentration
- Optimum Mental Clarity
- Enhanced Productivity & Work Output
- Decreased Stress
- Relaxed Attitude & Peace of Mind
- Positive Thinking & Attitude
- New Relationship to Food

Emotional Benefits
- Mood Uplift & Positive Outlook on life
- Long-lasting Emotional Balance
- Better Relationships and Interconnectedness
- Healing of Emotional Eating

Spiritual Benefits
- Equanimity
- Sense of Purpose
- Deep Inner Peace
- Connection to Others

7.   CONTRA-INDICATIONS AND POTENTIAL SIDE-EFFECTS

Cautions/ Contra-Indications

Anyone with a serious medical condition such as anemia, eating disorders, diabetes, kidney disease, autoimmune disease, cancer, terminal illnesses, certain genetic diseases, and other chronic conditions, who is considering going on a detox program/ diet should consult a qualified health professional and/or their medical doctor first and complete it under their supervision.

Pregnant women and nursing mothers should not go on a detox program/ diet as they need large amounts of food energy for the growing fetus/ infant. They should wait until after they give birth or stop lactating to start. They should never do a fast as they need to include as many healthy foods as possible into their daily regimen. Growing children fall into the same category and should not do a detox until after they stop growing. The raw vegan meal and the healthy meal program with proper additional super foods and using the detox kit can be completed under appropriate medical supervision.

The Detox programs/ diets offered as part of the Detox Goddess At Home Detox Kit are not intended for alcohol or drug detoxification, though they may help remove large amounts of toxins accumulated in the body of those suffering from substance-abuse. People suffering from serious addictions are advised to seek proper care to help with severe withdrawal symptoms. In-house detox programs are usually a better solution as the proper level of moral support can be provided to those in need.

If you are currently taking prescribed medication, these should never be discontinued or reduced without consulting the prescribing doctor and/ or your primary care provider first.

Side Effects

The following side effects are general in nature. They may or may not occur and do not specifically correspond to your experience while using a Detox Goddess At Home Detox Kit. For a more complete list of potential side-effects from detox, be sure to read below.

One of the most common side effects experienced within the first few days of starting a detox program/ diet is headaches/ migraines. This is mostly due to caffeine withdrawal or from other substances. This inconvenience can easily be avoided by following a short pre-detox regimen, which includes the gradual reduction of daily caffeine consumption (for a minimum of 3-5 days if you consume more than 2 cups of coffee a day.) or a slow wining of whatever other substance you may be using daily with an addictive component or attachment.

Another side effect might be irritability due to withdrawal from caffeine and the emotional component of attachment to specific foods, or solid food in general. Taking time off work to complete the cleanse, or choosing a holistic cleanse which offers many tools to deal with this type of issues, helps greatly minimize this type of stress. Check the Mindfulness program section of this manual (section 23) for more on that and how journaling and other mindfulness based activities can support your process.

Other side effects may include excessive diarrhea, which could lead to dehydration and electrolyte loss if left untreated. Constipation may occur if people consume excess fiber without also increasing their fluid intake.

Other possible side effects might include tiredness, skin breakout, weight loss, and hunger.

Any worsening of symptoms or new symptoms that occur during a detox program/ diet should prompt a visit to a qualified health care professional.

Following a detox program/ diet that omits animal products and does not provide adequate replacements for an extended period of time may result in nutrition deficiencies, particularly protein and calcium. The Detox programs provided as part of the Detox Goddess At Home Detox Kit offers superior nutrition through the inclusion of superfood and therefore do not constitute a high risk in this area.

8. DETOX KIT CONTENT

- Morning (AM) Detox Blend: 'Energy Rush' (1 x 5-day individual packet => take 1 serving daily for 5 days of detox)

- Midday (MID) Detox Blend: 'Immunity Boost' (1 x 5-day individual packet => take 1 serving daily for 5 days of detox)

- Evening (PM) Detox Blend: 'Repair & Anti-Inflammation' (1 x 5-day individual packet => take 1 serving daily for 5 days of detox)

- Daily Energy Brain Boosters (1 x 7-day individual sachet with 35 individual serving packets, i.e. 3/ day for 7 days of pre, post and detox)

- Nu-Detox Yoga Video including a 30-minute Detox Meditation (download available with free-trial (30 days) of the Detox Yoga Series on Stepflix at http://www.stepflix.com/#yoga/detox_yoga Use code ME23567 to redeem your 30-day free trial.)

- At Home Detox Kit Manual including a full guide to detoxification, 101 guide to juicing, detox recipes for juicing only detox, liquid only diet, raw vegan meal plan, or healthy meal program (e-version downloadable directly from our website at http://thedetoxco.com/portfolio/at-home-detox-kits/)

- Rebates on post-detox products & services (visit rebates center online at http://thedetoxco.com/portfolio/at-home-detox-kits/

9.   PRE-DETOX INSTRUCTIONS

The Detox Goddess 7-Day At Home Detox Kit has been designed to include products and instructions for 1 day of pre-detox and 1 day of post-detox, which is deemed the minimum time necessary in order to optimize a 5-day detox. If you can add an extra day of pre-detox and another one in post-detox, making it a 9-day detox program total, you will gain even more powerful results for very little extra work and it will make the transition in and out of your detox program feel like a breeze.

The supplies included in the Detox Goddess kit only cover the standard 7-day detox program. If you wish to add on a day (or more) of pre-detox, simply follow the same pre-detox instructions for the extra day+ without using the detox supplements provided for the 1-day of pre and post-detox. It will still prepare your body for optimum detox.

Guidelines relating to nutritional* intake for your day(s) of pre-detox are as follows:

OPTIONAL
(Optional) Upon awakening, drink a **fresh squeezed lemon tea** (squeeze 1/2 of a fresh organic lemon in hot alkaline Kangen** water.) If you suffer from constipation, this new addition to your daily food regimen will help you naturally relieve persistent constipation symptoms. If bowel movement remains sluggish, check the Detox Yoga Program section of this manual for specific information on what to do during Pre-Detox to help with this.

(Optional) If weight loss is one of your primary objectives for performing this detox program, or if you suffer from arthritis or other inflammatory conditions, we recommend that you add **Raw Apple Cider Vinegar***** to your daily diet regimen. This is also very good for people who suffer from heartburn. Take one teaspoon in 8 oz of fresh alkaline Kangen** water 3 times a day (breakfast/ lunch/ dinner.) If this formula is a little rough on your stomach, we recommend that you add a natural sweetener such as raw honey, raw agave syrup, black molasses, or stevia.

MORNING

Prepare your first **Energy Brain Booster** drink of the day by adding 3/4 of a teaspoon (3.6 g) of the Energy Brain Booster blend provided in your Detox Goddess 'At Home Detox Kit' to a glass of alkaline Kangen** water. Sweeten to taste using a natural sweetener (listed above) of your choice. You may also add 1/4 of a squeezed lemon for a fresher taste.

Wait at least 15 minutes after you've consumed your Energy Brain Booster drink before consuming anything else as this formula contains specific enzymes that will help you cleanse your digestive track and also optimize nutritional absorption.

For your first 'meal' of the day, we recommend a liquid meal **(juice or smoothie)** as a replacement for your **breakfast**. Refer to the Liquid Only Detox Program section of this manual for recipes of juices or smoothies. If you have opted for one of the non-liquid detox programs, you may consume some fresh low-glycemic fruits such as **berries**, a few **nuts****** and **seeds******* and some **fresh herb or fresh ginger tea**.

MID-DAY

Prepare your 2nd **Energy Brain Booster** drink of the day by adding 3/4 of a teaspoon (3.6 g) of the Energy Brain Booster blend provided in your Detox Goddess 'At Home Detox Kit' to a glass of alkaline Kangen** water. Sweeten to taste using the **natural**

sweetener (listed above) of your choice. You may also add 1/4 of a **squeezed lemon** for a fresher taste.

Wait at least 15 minutes after you've consumed your Energy Brain Booster drink before consuming anything else as this formula contains specific enzymes that will help you cleanse your digestive track and also optimize nutritional absorption.

For **lunch**, eat a light meal, such as a **mixed salad** or **brown-rice sushi**, or any other foods along the same **healthy** lines. You can find some recipes for inspiration in the Raw Vegan Meal Program and Healthy Meal Program (Vegetarian & Non-Vegetarian) - Guidelines sections of this manual.

EVENING

Prepare your 3rd **Energy Brain Booster** drink of the day by adding 3/4 of a teaspoon (3.6 g) of the Energy Brain Booster blend provided in your Detox Goddess 'At Home Detox Kit' to a glass of alkaline Kangen** water. Sweeten to taste using the natural sweetener (listed above) of your choice. You may also add 1/4 of a squeezed lemon for a fresher taste.

Wait at least 15 minutes after you've consumed your Energy Brain Booster drink before consuming anything else as this formula contains specific enzymes that will help you cleanse your digestive track and also optimize nutritional absorption.

For **dinner**, consume a **healthy soup**. Add a **small mixed salad** if you do not feel fully satiated (not full.)

Where possible, try to have **dinner before sundown** as the light of the sun (energy) is necessary for optimum digestion to take place.

ALL DAY

Avoid snacking throughout the day if you can, and leave at least 5-6 hours in between each meal to help with digestive rest. If you get a 'hunger' signal, **drink first instead**. Often times, we eat out of boredom, to fill an emotional need, or because we are dehydrated.

If you feel anxious about eating, ask your body if it is really hungry. (if you know the muscle testing technique, use it on yourself - it's really easy to do, or use a pendulum, to determine whether you are really hungry.) Pause, take 10 slow, deep breaths and see if you still feel hungry. If you are, then **choose a healthy snack** such a fresh carrots, a green apple, some berries, some nori sheets or dulse algae, or a few nuts or seeds.)

Remember that the normal size of your stomach is like your fist. So, try to keep your portions to that size where possible.

Volume-wise, **cut your food intake by at least 1/3**, i.e. take out 2 tablespoon(s) of your regular daily intake from all 3 meals. This will help shrink your stomach to its original size and also make the transition into your detox - especially if you have selected a liquid-only option, much smoother and emotionally tolerable.

Shifting to a **liquid-oriented diet** one day before the pre-detox day, i.e. using the same dietary recommendations listed above for an extra day (for a total of 2 days of pre-detox.) will make the transition into your detox easier and increase your detox benefits.

Avoid all processed foods and favor raw and fresh foods instead.

Avoid all caffeine including coffee, caffeinated teas and other beverages such as sodas. You may **consume decaffeinated tea**, preferably made from **fresh herbs and spices,** if desired.

Avoid all processed sugars and **use healthy natural sweetener alternatives** (listed above) instead.

Avoid all dairy products (milk, cheese, yogurt, etc.). Non-dairy milks such as almond, hemp, rice can be used instead.

Avoid oils. Replace them with **grated avocado, amino acids sauce, tamari, or apple cider vinegar and fresh sea salt** as condiments to your salads, soups, etc. You may also add or use **hemp, sesame or flax seeds.**

After the first few days, you may slowly start using small quantities of **extra virgin expeller-pressed olive or coconut oil. Cold pressed sesame oil** in very small amounts is ok too.

Favor **steamed, boiled, broiled, grilled** or **sautéed in water** with small amount of a first choice oil where possible. Avoid fried and heavily sautéed foods.

In addition to all the liquid drinks and foods you are already consuming, try to **drink about 8-10 glasses (8oz)** a day, or more if you were not already doing so on a regular basis and keep this as a healthy habit to improve digestion and smooth elimination, prevent dehydration and minimize your cravings for in-between meals snacking.

For additional guidelines, including the detox yoga program, alternative exercise program, as well as the mindfulness detox program, please refer to the relevant sections at the end of this manual.

For additional food guidelines for pre-detox with specific foods known for their highly detoxifying properties, refer to the

'Most Detoxifying Foods to eat in Pre- and Post-Detox' section of this book.

* All foods and drinks consumed should be organic where possible.
** If you do not own a Kangen water machine, we strongly suggest that you use the purest form of water you can find (preferably not bottled, or if so bottled in glass, and that you add purifying water drops****** such as http://amzn.com/B004IJHHL4 or MMS, an amazing destroyer of 99% pathogens which can be found at http://www.eden-health-products.com
*** Whether you choose the most renown Braggs brand, or find another choice, be sure that the Apple Cider Vinegar (ACV) you select is Raw and that it includes the mother of vinegar which contains all the nutrients necessary to give the desired benefits.
**** Best nuts - preferably in their raw or natural form, i.e. non-roasted and unsalted - to consume for maximum nutrition include; almonds, walnuts, pecans, and hazelnuts.
***** Best seeds - preferably in their raw or natural form, i.e. non-roasted and unsalted - to consume for maximum nutrition include; sunflower seeds and pumpkin seeds.
****** Please note that we are not associated with any of the companies that sell these products, and as such we are not gaining any benefits from the recommendations and suggestions we are making. Research and enjoy any and all suggestions at your own leisure.

10. POST-DETOX INSTRUCTIONS

The Detox Goddess 7-Day At Home Detox Kit was designed to include products and instructions for 1 day of pre-detox and 1 day of post-detox, which is deemed the minimum time necessary in order to optimize a 5-day detox. If you can add an extra day of pre-detox and another one in post-detox, making it a 9-day detox program total, you will gain even more powerful results for very little extra work and it will make the transition in and out of your detox program feel like a breeze. This will also optimize weight-loss objectives.

The supplies included in the Detox Goddess kit only cover the standard 7-day detox program. If you wish to add extra days of post-detox, simply follow the same post-detox instructions for the extra day+ without using the detox supplements provided for the 1-day of pre and post-detox. Post detox will help you move back into a more regular and solid-based food regimen, while keeping the benefits of new healthy eating habits and lightness of being.

Guidelines relating to nutritional* intake for your day(s) of post-detox are similar to pre-detox days as follows:

OPTIONAL

(Optional) Upon awakening, drink a **fresh squeezed lemon tea** (squeeze 1/2 of a fresh organic lemon in hot alkaline Kangen** water.) If you suffer from constipation, this new addition to your daily food regimen will help you naturally relieve persistent constipation symptoms. If bowel movement remains sluggish after the detox (which happens on rare occasions, especially if your body is not used to a new healthy liquid regimen), check the Detox Yoga Program section of this manual for specific information on what to do during Post-Detox to help with this.

(Optional) If weight loss was one of your primary objectives in performing this detox program, or if you suffer from arthritis or other inflammatory conditions, we recommend that you continue enjoying **Raw Apple Cider Vinegar (RACV)*** daily. This is also very good for people who suffer from heartburn. Take one teaspoon in 8 oz of fresh alkaline Kangen** water 3 times a day (breakfast/ lunch/ dinner.) If this formula is a little rough on your stomach, you may add a natural sweetener such as raw honey, raw agave syrup, black molasses, or stevia. There are no known side effects or contra-indications to the regular use of RACV, s super food, which provides a myriad of nutrients and healing properties for consumers of all ages.

MORNING

Just like in Pre-Detox, prepare your first **Energy Brain Booster** drink of the day by adding 3/4 of a teaspoon (3.6 g) of the Energy Brain Booster blend provided in your Detox Goddess 'At Home Detox Kit' to a glass of alkaline Kangen** water. Sweeten to taste using one of the natural sweeteners (listed above) of your choice. You may also add 1/4 of a fresh squeezed lemon for a fresher taste.

Wait at least 15 minutes after you've consumed your Energy Brain Booster drink before consuming anything else as this formula contains specific enzymes that will help you cleanse your digestive track and also optimize nutritional absorption.

For your first 'meal' of today, again we recommend a liquid meal **(juice or smoothie)** as a replacement for your **breakfast**. Refer to the Liquid Only Detox Program section of this manual for recipes of juices or smoothies. If you have opted for one of the non-liquid detox programs, you may consume some fresh low-glycemic fruits such as **berries**, a few **nuts****** and **seeds******* and some **fresh herb or fresh ginger tea**.

LUNCH

Right around lunch time, prepare your 2nd **Energy Brain Booster** drink of the day by adding 3/4 of a teaspoon (3.6 g) of the Energy Brain Booster blend provided in your Detox Goddess 'At Home Detox Kit' to a glass of alkaline Kangen** water. Sweeten to taste using one of the **natural sweeteners** (listed above) of your choice.

You may also add 1/4 of a **squeezed lemon** for a fresher taste.

Wait at least 15 minutes after you've consumed your Energy Brain Booster drink before consuming anything else as this formula contains specific enzymes that will help you cleanse your digestive track and also optimize nutritional absorption.

For **lunch**, you may stick to a liquid regimen if you wish to or simply eat a light meal similar to what you ate in Pre-Detox, i.e a **mixed salad** or **brown-rice sushi**, or any other foods along the same **healthy** lines are a great choice. You can find some recipes for inspiration in the Raw Vegan Meal Program and Healthy Meal Program (Vegetarian & Non-Vegetarian) - Guidelines sections of this manual.

EVENING

Around dinner time, prepare your 3rd **Energy Brain Booster** drink of the day by adding 3/4 of a teaspoon (3.6 g) of the Energy Brain Booster blend provided in your Detox Goddess 'At Home Detox Kit' to a glass of alkaline Kangen** water. Sweeten to taste using one of the natural sweeteners (listed above) of your choice. You may also add 1/4 of a squeezed lemon for a fresher taste.

Wait at least 15 minutes after you've consumed your Energy Brain Booster drink before consuming anything else as this formula contains specific enzymes that will help you cleanse your digestive track and also optimize nutritional absorption.

For **dinner**, stay with the same guidelines as in Pre-Detox and consume a **healthy soup**. Add a **small mixed salad** if you do not feel fully satiated (not full.)

Where possible, try to have **dinner before sundown,** as sunlight (energy) is necessary for optimum digestion to take place.

ALL DAY

Avoid snacking throughout the day if you can and leave at least 5-6 hours in between each meal to help with digestive rest. If you get a 'hunger' signal, **drink first instead**. Often times, we eat out of boredom, to fill an emotional need, or simply because we are dehydrated.

If you feel anxious about eating, ask your body if it is really hungry (if you know the muscle testing technique, use it on yourself - it's really easy to do, to determine whether you are really hungry. You may also use a pendulum.) Pause, take 10 deep breaths and see if you still feel hungry. If you are, then **choose a healthy snack** such a fresh carrots, a green apple, some berries, some nori sheets or dulse seaweed, or a few nuts or seeds.

Remember that the normal size of your stomach is the size of your fist. After a detox it may have shrunk a little too. So, try to keep your portions to that size where possible, or slowly building back up to the size of your fist.

Volume-wise, **slowly build your food intake back up** starting with 1/2 of the size of your regular meals before detox and slowly adding about 1 tablespoon of food at each meal (unless you were over-eating before your detox and are happy with smaller portion sizes now.) This will help slowly bring your stomach back to its original size and also make the transition out of your detox - especially if you have selected a liquid-only option, much smoother and let you keep the great benefits you gained during your detox.

Keeping a mainly **liquid-oriented diet** in the 1-2 days that follow your detox, i.e. using the same dietary recommendations listed above for an extra day (for a total of 2 days of post-detox.) will make the transition out of your detox easier and increase your detox benefits as well as optimize your weight-loss.

Avoid all processed foods and favor raw and fresh foods instead.

Avoid all caffeine including coffee, caffeinated teas and other beverages such as sodas. You may **consume decaffeinated tea**, preferably made from **fresh herbs and spices** if desired.

Avoid all processed sugars and **use healthy natural sweetener alternatives** (listed above) instead.

Avoid all dairy products (milk, cheese, yogurt, etc.)

Avoid oils and as a replacement use **grated avocado, amino acids sauce, tamari, or apple cider vinegar and fresh sea salt** as condiments to your salads, soups, etc. You may also add or use **hemp, sesame or flax seeds.**

After the first few days, you may slowly start using small quantities of **extra virgin expeller-pressed olive or coconut oil. Cold pressed sesame oil** in very small amounts is ok too.

In addition to all the liquid drinks and foods you are already consuming, try to **drink about 8-10 glasses (8oz)** a day, or more, if you were not already doing so on a regular basis and keep this as a healthy habit to improve digestion and smooth elimination, prevent dehydration and minimize your cravings for in-between meals snacking. This will help ensure that all the toxins and waste material that were released during your detox are completely flushed out of your system.

You may continue with your new healthy habits using all the food guidelines listed in the next section of this book to shift into healthier and more energy-oriented eating habits that will provide you with energy, dynamism, a strong immune system and many more health related benefits on all levels of your being (physical, mental, emotional, etc.)

For additional guidelines, including the detox yoga program, alternative exercise program, as well as the mindfulness detox program, please refer to the relevant sections at the end of this manual.

For additional food guidelines for post-detox with specific foods known for their highly detoxifying properties, refer to the 'Most Detoxifying Foods to eat in Pre- and Post-Detox' section of this book. Detox doesn't have to be something you do once in a while. Living a healthy life and eating a healthy diet can be a daily experience. We encourage you to continue with at least one liquid meal a day for optimum daily detoxification and to help minimize toxic and waste material build-up in your system.

ADDITIONAL

As a final note for your post-detox, if you want to continue to transition into a healthy diet and lifestyle use the following tips way after completely 1-2 days of post-detox.

Continue with as many liquid meals as possible for as long as you want or as a long-term choice, using a healthy source of protein to add to your juices and smoothies as listed in the pre-detox section of this manual in order to make sure that you do not develop any protein, vitamin, or mineral deficiencies. Remember to stay flexible, 'Never, Always, Forever' are words that limit us in the co-creation and manifestation of our deepest dreams and desires.

Where possible, continue taking a whole-food based supplement that will bring you all the vitamins and minerals that you need to live a balanced and healthy life. E3Live BrainOn is our preferred choice because it is a super food in itself, which contains easily absorbable vitamins, minerals, essential fatty acids, essential amino acids and enzymes that make all of these nutrients readily available. 1 serving of 1oz at least daily is a great way to start. For more on E3Live and all their products (which are the main staple of all our detox formulas, please visit them directly at www.e3live.com. Note that they have a 1-year unlimited satisfaction guarantee on all their products and a less than 1% return rate on all their products.)

Other whole food dietary supplements that you may consider continuing or starting to take after you complete your detox include; a good source of probiotics (or simply consuming a reasonable amount of fermented foods - as listed in the next section below, to get the same effect), a good source of additional enzymes (both probiotics and enzymes can also be purchased directly from E3Live), liquid chlorophyll with mint, GSE Extract, Vitamin E, vitamin D3 (min 5,000 IU).

If you drink alcohol, you may want to consider drinking artichoke tea (homemade or in-store) and milk thistle tea too as a preventative and repair tool for both the stomach and liver respectively.

Always favor steamed, boiled, broiled, grilled or sautéed in water with small amount of a first choice oil where possible. Avoid fried and heavily sautéed foods.

For non-liquid meals, Integrate as many raw foods as possible to your selections and avoid processed foods and sugar, pasteurized dairy products and excessive consumption of caffeinated beverages as much as possible.

Everything is about balance of course, so stay happy and content with what you eat while you continue to grow in awareness about the choices that you make diet-wise and how they affect your physical, mental and emotional states so that you can continue to make the healthiest and most logical choices for your long-term goals of health, overall wellbeing and longevity.

For an example of what your new food regimen could look like, along general lines;

Breakfast   (see relevant section of this book for recipes.)
- Fresh Green juice or smoothie of choice
Lunch   (see relevant section of this book for recipes.)
- Fresh juice or Smoothie
- or, Fresh Soup
- or/and, Fresh Salad

Dinner   (see relevant section of this book for recipes.)
- Fresh Soup
- or/+ Fresh Salad w/ seeds and grated avocado
- or/+ small quantities of Whole Grains (quinoa, brown rice, millet)
- or/and Fresh wild or organic high-quality fish (see section 9 below for a list of fish to consume safely on a regular basis)
- or/ and Fresh steamed, boiled or broiled vegetables

* All foods and drinks consumed should be organic where possible.
** If you do not own a Kangen water machine, we strongly suggest that you use the purest form of water you can find (preferably not bottled, or if so bottled in glass), and that you add purifying water drops****** such as http://amzn.com/B004IJHHL4 or MMS, an amazing destroyer of 99% pathogens which can be found at http://www.eden-health-products.com
*** Whether you choose the most renown Braggs brand, or find

another choice, be sure that the Apple Cider Vinegar (ACV) you select is Raw and that it includes the mother of vinegar which contains all the nutrients necessary to give the desired benefits.
**** Best nuts - preferably in their raw or natural form, i.e. non-roasted and unsalted - to consume for maximum nutrition include; almonds, walnuts, pecans, and hazelnuts.
***** Best seeds - preferably in their raw or natural form, i.e. non-roasted and unsalted - to consume for maximum nutrition include; sunflower seeds and pumpkin seeds.
****** Please note that we are not associated with any of the companies that sell these products, and as such we are not gaining any benefits from the recommendations and suggestions we are making. Research and enjoy any suggestions at your leisure.

11. MOST DETOXIFYING FOODS TO EAT IN PRE- AND POST-DETOX

In addition to the menus put together for you in the Raw Vegan Meals and Healthy Meals sections of this book, here is a list of the best foods to use in pre- and post-detox, or at any other time for optimum daily detox benefits. This gives you even more options to keep up with a tasty and healthy diet and helps you to achieve daily detox objectives to minimize your daily exposure to excess toxins and chemicals we inadvertently ingest through foods, water, air and the environment.

Where possible, consume the freshest foods, i.e. minimize your consumption of canned and processed foods, and limit frozen and dried foods too.

Eat organic whenever possible. Following is the list of the produce that must be eaten organic, no matter what, due to the different characteristics and factors that result in these fruits and vegetables being overloaded with pesticides and chemicals when grown conventionally (non organically.) Health experts have labeled it 'The Dirty Dozen' list due to the high toxicity of the fruits and vegetables on this list. I am adding Cilantro to the list as it is one of the main plants used in phyto-remediation of contaminated soil, and therefore it is a 'chemical'-loading machine that absorbs pesticides, chemicals and heavy metals present in the soil. I use organic cilantro in all my detox juices just for that reason, i.e. it binds the heavy metals and toxins released during the detox for safe elimination, and it tastes great too.

'MUST BE ORGANIC' LIST: 'THE DIRTY DOZEN'
The most pesticide-ridden produce items (classified by toxicity, 1 being the worst, and 12 the least worst) are;

FRUIT
1. Peaches (WORST)
2. Apples
5. Nectarines
6. Strawberries
7. Cherries
10. Imported Grapes
12. Pears

VEGETABLES
3. Sweet Bell Peppers
4. Celery
8. Kale
9. Lettuce
11. Carrots

Following is the list of produce that can be consumed in their inorganic form due to various factors - for the most part their thick outer skin, that make them least exposed to chemical and pesticide overload.

'NOT ORGANIC OK' LIST: **'THE SAFEST CONVENTIONAL BUYS'**
Produce with the least amount of pesticides is;

FRUIT
Cantaloupe
Kiwi
Watermelon
Pineapple
Mango
Grapefruit

VEGETABLES
Onions (BEST)
Sweet corn
Avocado
Asparagus
Sweet peas
Eggplant
Sweet potatoes
Mushrooms
Cabbage

The best way to use both lists to your advantage is as follows;
- If an item is on the actual top 12 'Dirty Dozen' list you should buy that produce in organic not conventional form. This will offer you the best protection from unnecessary exposure to pesticides and chemicals.
- If an item is on the 'Dirty Dozen' list, you need to make sure to also buy all derivatives of that produce in organic form. That means buying not only organic grapes and apples, but also buying organic apple juice, organic applesauce, organic raisins, organic grape jelly, etc.
- If you're looking to save cash on organics, the second list can help you choose which fruits and veggies are relatively safe to buy in

conventional form and are usually cheaper than organics. Saving money on lower-pesticide foods allows you to earmark more money for high pesticide foods.

In addition to the lists above, of additional concern are Genetically Modified Organisms (GMOs), which may pose a risk to your health in the L.T. The development of GMOs - that can resist pest and grow much faster than regular species, has not been tested long enough to be able to clearly assess the potential adverse consequences and side effects for humans consuming produce that has not been naturally grown. In light of these facts, it is better to abstain from consuming them and remain safe in that regard. Following are a few simple tips to avoid GMOs.

1.   Buy Organic—Certified products that carry the USDA or '100% organic' label. Organic products cannot intentionally include any GMO ingredients.
2.   Also, check for "Non-GMO Project" verified seals wherever possible for an even safer option.
3.   When purchasing conventional produce, avoid at-risk ingredients such as soybeans, corn, canola, cottonseed and sugar from sugar beets. More than 93% of these ingredients are known to be grown as GMOs in the U.S.
4.   Other produce at risk include; most Hawaiian papaya, a small volume of zucchini and yellow squash, sugar (from U.S. origin and NOT pure cane sugar, as the source is often partly sugar beets.)
5.   Finally, avoid conventional dairy products that may originate from cows injected with GM bovine growth hormone (growth hormone is associated with genetic mutation and the development of tumors.) Look for labels stating No rBGH, rBST, or artificial hormones.

Now that we've identified certain qualities of foods that

should be avoided, let's look at where our focus should be to gain optimum daily detox benefits. This is a non-exhaustive list of foods and super foods with the highest nutrient content and most detoxifying in nature.

VEGETABLES
- All dark leafy and cruciferous greens including but not limited to;
* kale
* collard greens
* broccoli
* turnip greens
* swiss chard
* spinach
*mustard greens
* red and green leaf and romaine lettuce
* cabbage
* cauliflower
- dandelion
- artichoke
- green asparagus
- leeks
- beet greens
- green beans
- sweet and sugar snap peas
- baby spinach
- baby kale
- arugula
- romaine lettuce
- celery
- fennel
- cucumber
- all sprouts (sunflower, pea green, broccoli, alfalfa, mung beans, garbanzo beans, adzuki beans, black eyed peas, etc.)

HERBS, ROOTS & SPICES

- fresh cilantro
- fresh parsley
- fresh mint
- fresh basil
- fresh thyme
- curcumin/ turmeric
- cayenne pepper
- fresh ginger
- wheatgrass shot (daily if possible) (note: wheatgrass contains over 123 vitamins and minerals and is a full body healer, powerful health regenerator all of itself.)

FRUIT
- avocado
- lemon & lime
- green apples
- all berries (acai berries, blueberries, raspberries, strawberries, Goji berries, cranberries, etc.)
- rhubarb
- papaya (for digestion)
- grapefruit (for slimming effect)
- pineapple (in small volumes to cut grease/ fat in the body)

NUTS & SEEDS & ALL RAW BUTTERS
- raw almonds
- raw walnuts
- raw pecans
- raw hazelnut
- raw pumpkin seeds
- raw sunflower seeds
- sesame seeds (especially black)
- hemp seeds
- chia seeds
- flax seeds (both whole and freshly ground)

- All raw butters derived from the nuts and seeds listed above

OILS
- cold pressed extra virgin olive oil
- cold pressed extra virgin coconut oil
- cold pressed sesame oil (small volume)
- raw tahini (small volume)

GRAINS & CEREALS
- sprouted quinoa
- sprouted brown rice
- other non-wheat sprouted grains of choice (rye, kalmut, etc.)

BEANS & LEGUMES
- sprouted lentils
- sprouted garbanzo beans
- black beans
- adzuki beans
- other high-nutrient, high fiber legumes of choice (kidney beans, lima beans, pinto beans, navy beans, etc.)

SEA VEGETABLES
- kombu
- kelp
- dulse
- nori
- wakame
- agar-agar
- etc.

FERMENTED FOODS
(good source of natural probiotics and enzymes.)
- miso (preferably not of soybean origin or 100% organic)
- tempeh

- sauerkraut
- fermented beet shreds
- kim chi (spicy Korean cabbage mix)
- umeboshi plums (Japanese dried plums)
- kombucha tea (preferably non-alcoholic)
- kefir (especially from coconut water and goat's milk)
- some cultured milk and derived milk products
- dark chocolate
- pickles
- olives
- etc.

FISH*
Only wild or organic farm raised. Examples of some of the healthiest fish to eat include;
- Albacore tuna (troll- or pole-caught, from the U.S. or British Columbia)
- salmon (wild-caught, Alaska)
- oysters (farmed), which is also known for its amazing aphrodisiac virtues
- sardines, Pacific (wild-caught)
- rainbow trout (farmed)
- freshwater Coho salmon (farmed in tank systems, from the U.S.)

Due to the increasing concern relating to high mercury (a highly health-hazardous heavy metal) levels found in fish, be sure to check for a full list of fish to consume and how often at the end of this section. For full guidelines on frequency of consumption of all fish, visit http://www.nrdc.org/health/effects/mercury/guide.asp.)

BEVERAGES
- alkaline water (preferably Kangen alkaline water)
- bancha tea
- fresh green tea

- kombucha (preferably non-alcoholic)
- iodine water (from reliable sources amd in the form of nascent iodine.)

SWEETENERS
- raw manuka honey (UMF 16 and up) (do not put in heated beverage as it will destroy all the beneficial nutrients)
- raw agave syrup
- blackstrap molasses
- raw brown sugar
- stevia
- brown rice syrup
- maple syrup grade AA light amber

SUPERGREEN SUPER FOODS
The super foods listed below are a great addition to your daily diet for optimum nutrition, immune function, overall health and to support daily detox objectives. They also have a high-protein content in an easily digestible form (available as amino acids from which human protein can be built.)

- blue-green algae (E3Live being the only one available in 'alive' frozen form)
- de-walled chlorella
- spirulina
- wheatgrass
- barley grass
- etc.

For more on foods and super foods to incorporate into your daily food regimen, please visit our website at http://thedetoxco.com/superfoods-for-life/

* FISH

The list of fish and frequency of consumption below has been extracted from the FRDC*** guide. It applies to fish caught and sold commercially and relates to 6 oz servings for a person of 130lb/ 60kg. For information about fish you catch yourself, check for advisories in your state.

FISH with the LEAST MERCURY that can be enjoyed **liberally**;
(Less than 0.09 parts per million - Mercury.)
-Anchovies
- Butterfish
- Catfish
- Clam
- Crab (Domestic)
- Crawfish/Crayfish
- Croaker (Atlantic)
- Flounder*
- Haddock (Atlantic)*
- Hake
- Herring
- Mackerel (N. Atlantic, Chub)
- Mullet
- Oyster
- Perch (Ocean)
- Plaice
- Pollock
- Salmon (canned)**
- Salmon (fresh)**
- Sardine
- Scallop*
- Shad (American)
- Shrimp*
- Sole (Pacific)
- Squid (Calamari)
- Tilapia

- Trout (freshwater)
- Whitefish
- Whiting

FISH with MODERATE MERCURY that you should eat **no more than six servings per month**;
(From 0.09 to 0.29 parts per million - Mercury)
- Bass (Striped, Black)
- Carp
- Cod (Alaskan)*
- Croaker (White Pacific)
- Halibut (Atlantic)*
- Halibut (Pacific)
- Jacksmelt (Silverside)
- Lobster
- Mahi Mahi
- Monkfish*
- Perch (freshwater)
- Sablefish
- Skate*
- Snapper*
- Tuna (canned chunk light)
- Tuna (Skipjack)*
- Weakfish (Sea Trout)

FISH with HIGH MERCURY that you should eat **no more than three servings per month**;
(From 0.3 to 0.49 parts per million - Mercury)
- Bluefish
- Grouper*
- Mackerel (Spanish, Gulf)
- Sea Bass (Chilean)*
- Tuna (canned Albacore)
- Tuna (Yellowfin)*

FISH with the HIGHEST MERCURY that you should **avoid** eating
altogether;
 (More than .5 parts per million - Mercury)
- Mackerel (King)
- Marlin*
- Orange Roughy*
- Shark*
- Swordfish*
- Tilefish*
- Tuna (Bigeye, Ahi)*

* These fish are also perilously low in numbers or are caught using
environmentally destructive methods.
** Farmed Salmon may contain PCB's, i.e. chemicals with serious
long-term health effects.
Sources for NRDC's guide: The data for this guide to mercury in fish
comes from two federal agencies: the Food and Drug
Administration, which tests fish for mercury, and the Environmental
Protection Agency, which determines mercury levels that it considers
safe for women of childbearing age.

12. DETOX INSTRUCTIONS

Now that you have completed one or two days of pre-detox,
you are ready to start with your detox program. By reducing
volumes, switching to a more liquid-based regimen, eating more
raw and unprocessed foods, beginning to boost your immunity and
increase energy levels through the use of super foods and
increasing your water intake, you have prepared your body for
optimum detoxification and minimum anxiety in relation to
emotional eating. That said, some people who have strong
emotional attachment to certain, or/ and solid foods in general,
may sill experience some level of discomfort and anxiety in the first

2, or even up to the 3rd day of detox but this is extremely rare if you prepare your body and mind by following a pre-detox regimen. By day 3, all feelings of emotional hunger should have disappeared, even for those on the Juice Only Detox Program. If you are experiencing any of these symptoms, please refer to the Optional Mindfulness Detox Program for specific instructions on how to deal with anxiety over food cravings. Breath-work and meditation are particularly effective to deal with emotional eating and withdrawal symptoms. It is as simple as taking 10 slow, deep breaths anytime you feel the 'eating' panic attack building up. Tapping, also described under the Mindfulness Program, is another powerful technique to release such stress.

Your Goddess Detox At-Home Kit gives you 4 options in terms of the food regimen you select for your detox. In all cases, you will experience detoxification benefits. That said, the liquid-based programs offer you the most benefits. Still, we give the options of following a healthy food plan during a detox because we believe that a certain level of detox is better than no detox at all. And in detox like with anything else in life, there are levels. For most people, it is completely unrealistic to go right from a heavily processed diet to a juice-only cleanse. An athlete doesn't run 100 meters in under 10 seconds without some preliminary steps and training. So, go easy on yourself. Take steps towards a realistic and equally rewarding detoxification program that will result in long lasting healthy habits.

Following are the 4 main detox programs you can follow using your Detox Goddess At-Home Detox Kit;

1. Juice Only Program - Guidelines
2. Liquid Only Program (Juice & Smoothie) - Guidelines
3. Raw Vegan Meal Program - Guidelines
4. Healthy Meal Program (Vegetarian & Non-Vegetarian) - Guidelines

Here are general food guidelines that apply to all 4 programs. For individual guidelines/ recipes, with the only element that varies from one detox program to another being the food you consume, please refer to the next 4 sections of this book. Some of these guidelines are the same as the ones you will be using in the pre- and post-detox phases of your detox.

OPTIONAL

(Optional) Upon awakening, drink a **fresh squeezed lemon tea** (squeeze 1/2 of a fresh organic lemon in hot alkaline Kangen** water.) If you suffer from constipation, this new addition to your daily food regimen will help you naturally relieve persistent constipation symptoms. If bowel movement remains sluggish after the detox (this happens on rare occasions especially if your body is not used to a new healthy liquid regimen), check the Detox Yoga Program section of this manual for specific information on what to do during Post-Detox to help with this.

(Optional) If weight loss is one of your primary objectives in performing this detox program, or if you suffer from arthritis or other inflammatory conditions, we recommend that you consume **Raw Apple Cider Vinegar (RACV)*** daily. This is also very good for people who suffer from heartburn. Take one teaspoon in 8 oz of fresh alkaline Kangen** water 3 times a day (breakfast/ lunch/ dinner.) If this formula is a little rough on your stomach, simply add a natural sweetener such as raw honey, raw agave syrup, black molasses, or stevia. There are no known side-effects or contra-indications to the regular use of RACV, a super food which provides myriads of nutrients and healing properties for all consumers.

MORNING

Just like in Pre-Detox, prepare your first **Energy Brain Booster** drink of the day by adding 3/4 of a teaspoon (3.6 g) of the Energy Brain Booster blend provided in your Detox Goddess 'At Home Detox Kit' to a glass of alkaline Kangen** water. Sweeten to taste using one of the natural sweeteners (listed above) of your choice. You may also add 1/4 of a squeezed lemon for a fresher taste.

Wait at least 15 minutes after you've consumed your Energy Brain Booster drink before consuming anything else as this formula contains specific enzymes that will help you cleanse your digestive track and also optimize nutritional absorption.

For your first 'meal' of the day, refer to the appropriate section of this book for the detox program you've selected to find your day-to-day 'food' program.

MID-DAY

Right around lunch time, prepare your 2nd **Energy Brain Booster** drink of the day by adding 3/4 of a teaspoon (3.6 g) of the Energy Brain Booster blend provided in your Detox Goddess 'At Home Detox Kit' to a glass of alkaline Kangen** water. Sweeten to taste using one of the **natural sweeteners** (listed above) of your choice. You may also add 1/4 of a **squeezed lemon** for a fresher taste.

Wait at least 15 minutes after you've consumed your Energy Brain Booster drink before consuming anything else as this formula contains specific enzymes that will help you cleanse your digestive track and also optimize nutritional absorption.

For 'lunch', refer to the appropriate section of this book for the detox program you've selected to find your day-to-day 'food' program.

Around dinner time, prepare your 3rd **Energy Brain Booster** drink of the day by adding 3/4 of a teaspoon (3.6 g) of the Energy Brain Booster blend provided in your Detox Goddess 'At Home Detox Kit' to a glass of alkaline Kangen** water. Sweeten to taste using one of the natural sweeteners (listed above) of your choice. You may also add 1/4 of a squeezed lemon for a fresher taste.

Wait at least 15 minutes after you've consumed your Energy Brain Booster drink before consuming anything else as this formula contains specific enzymes that will help you cleanse your digestive track and also optimize nutritional absorption.

EVENING

For 'dinner', refer to the appropriate section of this book for the detox program you've selected to find your day-to-day 'food' program.

Where possible, try to have **'dinner' before sundown,** as sunlight (energy) is necessary for optimum digestion to take place.

Avoid snacking throughout the day if you can and leave at least 5-6 hours in between each meal to help with digestive rest. If you get a 'hunger' signal, **drink first instead**. Often times, we eat out of boredom, to fill an emotional need, or simply because we are dehydrated.

If you feel anxious about eating, ask your body if it is really hungry (if you know the muscle testing technique, use it on yourself - it's really easy to do, to determine whether you are really hungry.) Pause, take 10 deep breaths and see if you still feel hungry. If you are, **choose a healthy snack,** such a fresh carrots, a green apple, some berries, or a few nuts**** or seeds******.
In addition to all the liquid drinks and foods you are already

consuming, try to **drink about 8-10 glasses (8oz)** a day, or more if you were not already doing so on a regular basis and keep this as a healthy habit to improve digestion and smooth elimination, prevent dehydration and minimize your cravings for in-between meals snacking. This will help ensure that all the toxins and waste material that were released during your detox are completely flushed out of your system.

NON-LIQUID PROGRAMS ONLY

The following guidelines only apply to customers who have selected a non-liquid healthy meal plan. Please follow as directed below;

Important note: Customers who selected the non-liquid healthy meal plan option should use the detox powder mixes in their daily boosters. For all 3 times of the day where you take the boosters, you can add the detox powder mixes that correspond to that time of the day. Conversely, you may opt to add a green and light juice to your meal plan and use the detox powder mix formulas in those and in addition to the boosters you are already consuming.

Remember that the normal size of your stomach is the size of your fist and during detox you should try to keep your food portion to the size of your fist or smaller at any one seating.

Volume-wise, during the detox, you can choose to slowly decrease the size of your meals if you are comfortable doing so, using the same rule you used in pre-detox, i.e. reducing meal size by 1 tablespoon of food at each meal.

Avoid all processed foods and favor raw and fresh foods instead as per the specific menu guidelines that apply to your detox program.

Avoid all caffeine including coffee, caffeinated teas and other beverages such as sodas. You may **consume decaffeinated tea**, preferably made from **fresh herbs and spices** if desired.

Avoid all processed sugars and **use healthy natural sweetener alternatives** (listed above) instead. If you are trying to lose weight, cut out as many sweeteners as possible.

Avoid all dairy products (milk, cheese, yogurt, etc.)

Avoid oils and replace them with **grated avocado, amino acids sauce, tamari, or raw apple cider vinegar and fresh sea salt** as condiments to your salads, soups, etc. You may also add or use **hemp, sesame or flax seeds.**

All guidelines relating to the exercise and mindfulness programs you wish to follow during your detox program are included in the relevant sections of this book under 'Optional Exercise Program' and 'Optional Additional Mindfulness Program.'

* All foods and drinks consumed should always be organic where possible.
** If you do not own a Kangen water machine, we strongly suggest that you use the purest form of water you can find (preferably not bottled, or if so bottled in glass, and that you add purifying water drops**** such as http://amzn.com/B004IJHHL4 or MMS, an amazing destroyer of 99% pathogens which can be found at http://www.eden-health-products.com
*** Whether you choose the most renown Braggs brand, or find another choice, be sure that the Apple Cider Vinegar (ACV) you select is Raw and that it includes the mother of vinegar which contains all the nutrients necessary to give the desired benefits.
**** Best nuts - preferably in their raw or natural form, i.e. non-roasted and unsalted - to consume for maximum nutrition include;

almonds, walnuts, pecans, and hazelnuts.

***** Best seeds - preferably in their raw or natural form, i.e. non-roasted and unsalted - to consume for maximum nutrition include; sunflower seeds and pumpkin seeds.

13. JUICE ONLY PROGRAM - GUIDELINES

Following are recipes for you to use during your 7-day cleanse.

Day 1 and Day 7, are pre- and post-detox days respectively, but you may choose to incorporate a juice from this menu during those days since it is advisable to start shifting from solid to more liquid foods in pre-detox and to transition smoothly back into solid in post-detox. Thought they are classified by day, you can choose to rearrange your menu however you like and repeat juices that are particularly appealing to you as long as you keep at least one Green juice (labeled as such) a day. All ingredients in your juices should be organic as you are looking to detoxify and minimize further toxic exposure to your system. Keep in mind, that the body grows healthier and stronger, and the mind more flexible, when food intake is fresh and varied.

For juicing, I highly recommend using the Omega j8006 Nutrition Center Masticating Juicer, or the Breville JE98XL Juice Fountain Plus 850-Watt Juice Extractor if your budget is limited.

Day 2 -

Energy Rush I (Green Juice)
- Celery (4 stalks)
- Spinach (1/2 bunch)
- Apples* (1-2**)
- Cilantro (1/4 bunch)

- Lemon (1/2)

Power Flush (Green Juice)
- Cucumber (1)
- Apples* (1-2**)
- Ginger (about 1/4 root - 2")***
- Mint (1/4 bunch)
- Lemon (1/2)

Repair Miracle I
- Beet (1 small)
- Carrots (3-4 large)
- Apple* (1/2)
- Parsley (1/4 bunch)
- Ginger (about 1/4 root - 2")***
- Lemon (1/2)

Day 3 -

Slim Twist
- Grapefruit (1)
- Oranges (2)
- Lime (1)
- Lemon (1)

Radical Flush (Green Juice)
- Cucumber (1)
- Broccoli (1 head)
- Apples* (1-2**)
- Cilantro (1/4 bunch)
- Lemon (1/2)

Repair miracle II
- Beet (2 smalls)

- Carrots (3-4 large)
- Parsley (1/4 bunch)
- Ginger (about 1/4 root - 2")***
- Lemon (1/2)

Day 4 -

Fresh Start
- Green Apples (4)
- Ginger (about 1/4 root - 2")***
- Lemon (1/2)
Immunity Boost
- Carrots (3-4 large)
- Oranges (2)
- Ginger (about 1/4 root - 2")***
- Lemon (1/2)

Sole Comfort I
- Beet (1 small)
- Carrots (3-4 large)
- Cucumber (1/2)
- Parsley (1/4 bunch)
- Ginger (about 1/4 root - 2")***
- Lemon (1/2)

Day 5 -

Energy Rush II (Green Juice)
- Celery (4 stalks)
- Dandelion (1/2 bunch)
- Apples* (1-2**)
- Cilantro (1/4 bunch)
- Lemon (1/2)

Power Flush (Green Juice)
- Cucumber (1)
- Apples* (1-2**)
- Ginger (about 1/4 root - 2")***
- Mint (1/4 bunch)
- Lemon (1/2)

Sole Comfort II
- Beet (1 small)
- Carrots (3-4 large)
- Orange (1)
- Ginger (about 1/4 root - 2")***
- Lemon (1/2)

Day 6 -

Energy Rush III (Green Juice)
- Celery (4 stalks)
- Kale (1/2 bunch)
- Apples* (1-2**)
- Cilantro (1/4 bunch)
- Lemon (1/2)

Green Cooler (Green Juice)
- Fresh Coconut Water (min 14 oz)
- Sunflower Seed Sprouts (1/4 bunch)
- Cilantro (1/4 bunch)
- Mint (1/4 bunch)
- Ginger (about 1/4 root - 2")***

Repair Miracle I
- Beet (1 small)
- Carrots (3-4 large)
- Apple* (1/2)

- Parsley (1/4 bunch)
- Ginger (about 1/4 root - 2")***
- Lemon (1/2)

* Green Apples preferred (if you have a sweet tooth, use Fuji apples as an alternative.)
** If you have a sweet tooth, use two apples to sweeten your green juices, preferably green apples. If not, stick to 1 or 1.5 apples.
*** If you are a regular ginger user/ lover, you can add more ginger to taste than what is recommended above.

14. LIQUID ONLY PROGRAM (JUICE & SMOOTHIE) - GUIDELINES

If weight-loss is not one of your primary objectives for doing a detox and you enjoy the taste of sweetness and smoothies, you may opt for the Liquid Only Program, which incorporates both juices and smoothies. Use any of the juices you wish to from the Juices Only program and then add any of the smoothies listed below. You may substitute a juice for a smoothie, or two juices for two smoothies, or also add smoothies to the Juices Only program if you feel the need for more nutrition (athletes in training or people who are currently underweight). Just be sure to keep at least one Green Juice a day.

Also, if you are worried about weight-loss, you may use a protein powder mix of your choice. We recommend using super foods such as E3Live Blue-Green Algae, de-walled Chlorella, Spirulina, or a blend of these. Alternatively, hemp protein, pea protein and barley protein, or a combination of super greens protein are also a good choice.
Smoothies require a blender. I highly recommend the use of a Vitamix, or a Nutri-bullet, if your budget is more limited.
As with the Juice Only Program, each day you will consume 3

liquid meals. Combinations could be; 1 Green Juice & 2 Smoothies, 1 Juice, 1 Juice and 1 Smoothies, etc.

Following are recipes for great-tasting, nutrient-dense smoothies for use as substitute or addition to the juices offered in the Juice Only Program;

Day 2 -

Slim Avocado Delight (Green smoothie)
- Avocado (1/2)
- Green Apple (1)
- Pineapple (1/8)
- Spinach (1/2 bunch)
- Lemon (1)
- Ice (1/2 cup*)

Raw Acai Bowl
- Banana (1)
- Acai berries (1 frozen)
- Ice (1/2 cup*)

Day 3 -

Sweet Almond Green (Green Smoothie)
-Banana (1)
- Pear (1)
- Raw Almonds (10-15)
- Dates (1-2)
- Spinach (1/2 bunch)
- Ice (1/2 cup*)

Raw Cacao Bliss
- Avocado (1/2)

- Banana (1)
- Fresh Young Coconut Flesh or Unsweetened Coconut Flakes (1/4 coconut or a few handfuls of flakes)
- Raw Cacao Powder (2 teaspoons)

Day 4 -

Raw Green Berry Bliss
- Avocado (1/2)
- Banana (1)
- Blueberries (4 oz)
- Spinach (1/2 bunch)
- Ice (1/2 cup*)

Raw Banana Avocado Bliss
- Avocado (1/2)
- Banana (1)
- Ground Flax Seeds (2 teaspoons)
- Chia Seeds (2 teaspoons)
- Ice (1/2 cup*)

Day 5 -

Raw Almond Strawberry Bliss
- Avocado (1/2)
- Banana (1)
- Strawberries (4 oz)
- Spinach (1/2 bunch)
- Raw Almonds (10-15)
- Ice (1/2 cup*)

Raw Coco-Pineapple Bliss
- Banana (1)
- Pineapple (1/8)

- Coconut Milk (4 oz)
- Maca Powder (2 teaspoons)
- Chia seeds (2 teaspoons)
- Ice (1/2 cup*)

Day 6 -

Papaya-Orange Tropical Bliss
- Banana (1)
- Papaya (1/8)
- Orange (1)
- Cinnamon (2 teaspoon)
- Dates (1-2)
- Ice (1/2 cup*)

Raw Cacao Maca Bliss
- Avocado (1/2)
- Raw Almonds (10-15)
- Fresh Young Coconut Flesh or Unsweetened Coconut Flakes (1/4 coconut or a few handfuls of flakes)
- Raw Cacao (2 teaspoons)
- Maca Powder (2 teaspoons)
- Flax seeds (2 teaspoons)
- Ice (1/2 cup*)

* If you want to give your smoothie a more watery consistency, add up to 1 cup of ice. This might yield a little more than a 16oz smoothie.

15. RAW VEGAN MEAL PROGRAM - GUIDELINES

If you opted for the 7-day Raw Vegan Meal Program, you have the option to break down the 7 days into 1 day of pre-detox, 1 day of post-detox (using the specific guidelines provided in the appropriate sections of this manual) and follow the instructions and recipes for the Raw Vegan Meal Program for the remaining 5 days. Alternately, you may follow the plan for the entire 7-day period. You may also choose to extend the Raw Vegan Meal Program for as long as you'd like after the 7-day period has ended, and eventually integrate the nutritious foods and super foods you used during your detox program into your daily food regimen for optimum daily detox, health and overall wellbeing.

Following are sample recipes you may want to use during your 7-day Raw Vegan Meal Program. If time is an issue for you and you have the budget for it, you can also hire a raw vegan chef. As another option, you may use recipes from any Raw Food cookbook at your own discretion.

Remember that you can integrate any of the juices listed in the Juice Only Detox Program into your daily detox program if you wish to as long as your primary objective for detoxing is not weigh-loss (since the addition of the juices will slightly increase your caloric intake.) You may also replace some of the raw vegan meals with juices or smoothies. The combinations and options are endless. The only important rule to follow if for you to consume your detox mixes, booster and juice/ smoothie mixes daily, no matter how you wish to integrate them into your routine. See specific instructions under the appropriate sections that cover those detox supplements and detox instructions.

We have classified the meals by day, but you can rearrange your menu however you like and repeat meals that are particularly appealing to you as long as you vary the meals a little for fun, diversity and optimum nutrition. All ingredients in your meals should be organic and as fresh as possible in order to optimize detoxification and minimize further toxic exposure to your system.
Interestingly enough the emphasis is primarily about what not

to eat rather than what to eat. Refer to the pre- and post-detox guidelines where we listed all the foods you should avoid in those times. This also applies for detox.

Day 1 -

Breakfast
- mixed berries (raspberries, blueberries, strawberries) (1/2 cup)
- raw almond butter (4 tsp) on 1/2 gluten-free wrap or apple (1/2)
- wheatgrass shot (1-2 oz)

Lunch
- raw cream of celery soup (6 oz)
- green salad with arugula, spinach, dandelion, baby greens (8 oz)
- sunflower seeds (4 tsp)
- grated avocado (1/2)
- chia seeds (2 tsp)
- balsamic vinegar (2 tsp)
- celtic sea salt (optional)
- fresh ginger tea (1/4 root of fresh sliced ginger boiled and then simmered in water for 10-15 mms)

Dinner
- freshly made hummus (4-6 oz)
- fresh cucumber slices & mini carrots (for the hummus - approx. 5-10 of each)
- side of fresh Kim chi or sauerkraut (4 tsp)
- fresh chamomile leaves tea (10 leaves boiled + simmered in water for 10-15 mms) - add natural sweetener if necessary (1/2 tsp)

Day 2 -

Breakfast
- green juice (2 green apples, 1/4 bunch of kale, 1/4 bunch of spinach, 1 celery stalk, 1/4 bunch of cilantro, 1/4 root of ginger,

1/4 lemon juice)
- 1/4 pomegranate fruit (1/4 cup)
- wheatgrass shot (1-2 oz)

Lunch
- sprouted herb & almond pate (4 oz)
- fresh celery & carrots (for the pate - approx. 5 of each)
- fresh greens & herbs (baby spinach & kale, cilantro, dill) (4 oz)
- fresh tahini (1tbsp)
- apple cider vinegar (1 tsp)
- celtic sea salt (optional)
- fresh mint tea (1/2 bunch of fresh mint leaves boiled + simmered in water for 10-15 mms) - add natural sweetener if desired (1/2 tsp)

Dinner
- raw gazpacho soup w/ fresh cilantro (4 oz)
- 1/2 avocado w/ gomashio seasoning (1 tsp), umeboshi vinegar (1 tsp) , and black sesame seeds (1 tsp)
- fresh ginger tea (1/4 root of fresh sliced ginger boiled + simmered in water for 10-15 mms) - add natural sweetener if desired (1/2 tsp)

Day 3 -

Breakfast
- mixed berries (raspberries, blueberries, strawberries) (1/3 cup)
- raw hemp butter (3 tsp) on 1/3 gluten-free wrap or apple (1/3)
- wheatgrass shot (1-2 oz)

Lunch
- raw vegan coleslaw (4 oz)
- green salad with arugula, spinach, dandelion, baby greens (6 oz)
- raw pumpkin seeds (2 tsp)
- grated avocado (1/3)
- chia seeds (1 tsp)
- balsamic vinegar (1 tsp)
- pink himalayan sea salt (optional)

- 1 fresh ginger shot (1-2 oz)

Dinner
- fresh veggie sushi w/ vegetables - avocado, shredded carrots, beets, zucchini and cucumber inside seaweed wrappings (4-6 pcs)
- fresh Wakame seaweed salad (4 oz)
- side of fresh kimchi or sauerkraut (3 tsp)
- fresh parsley tea (1/4 bunch of fresh parsley boiled + simmered in water for 15-20 mms)- add natural sweetener if necessary (1/2 tsp)

Day 4 –

Breakfast
- Enlivening smoothie (3 peeled carrots, 1/2 cucumber, 2 oranges, 1 mandarin, 1/2 lemon, 1/4 root of ginger, 10-15 ice-cubes)
- wheatgrass shot (1-2 oz)

Lunch
- raw green pea soup (4 oz)
- endives/ chicory & sliced almonds salad (4 oz)
- hemp seeds (1 tbsp)
- balsamic vinegar (1 tsp)
- grated avocado (1/4)
- celtic sea salt (optional)

Dinner
- freshly made raw Baba Ganoush (4 oz)
- fresh broccoli florets & snap peas (for the Baba Ganoush dip - approx. 5 of each)
- side of fresh kimchi or sauerkraut (2 tsp)
- fresh ginger tea (1/4 root of fresh sliced ginger boiled + simmered in water for 10-15 mms) - add natural sweetener if desired (1/2 tsp)

Day 5 -

Breakfast

- mixed berries (raspberries, blueberries, strawberries) (1/4 cup)
- raw almond butter (2 tsp) on 1/4 gluten-free wrap or apple (1/4)
- wheatgrass shot (1-2 oz)

Lunch
- raw cream of cucumber soup (3-4 oz)
- fresh kale salad (4 oz)
- fresh minced garlic (1-2 cloves)
- tahini (1 tsp)
- raw apple cider vinegar (1tsp)
- hemp seeds (2 tsp)
- balsamic vinegar (2 tsp)
- celtic sea salt (optional)
- fresh ginger shot (1-2 oz)

Dinner
- freshly made Guacamole (3-4 oz)
- fresh zucchini sticks, broccoli, and red pepper slices cucumber
slices (for the guacamole - approx. 3-4 of each)
- fresh rehydrated* almonds and walnuts (10-15 total)
- fresh parsley tea (1/4 bunch of fresh parsley boiled + simmered in
water for 15-20 mms) - add natural sweetener if necessary (1/2 tsp)

Day 6 -

Breakfast
- Greenie smoothie (1/2 banana, 1/8 pineapple, 1/2 avocado,
1/4 bunch of spinach, 1 tsp hemp seed, 5-10 ice cubes)
- wheatgrass shot (1-2 oz)

Lunch
- hemp beet soup (3-4 oz)
- fresh cilantro (1/8 bunch)
- green beans salad (4 oz)
- sliced almonds (2 tbsp)
- chia seeds (1 tsp)

- balsamic vinegar (2 tsp)
- celtic sea salt (optional)
- ginger shot (1-2 oz)

Dinner
- fresh veggies in nori seaweed wrap (vegetables of choice: avocado, shredded beet, zucchini, and carrots, broccoli and sunflower sprouts)
- fresh tahini for the wrap (1 tbsp)
- fresh gomashio seasoning (1 tsp)
- fresh coconut amino acids (1 tsp)
- raw blended tomato and basil soup (3 oz)

Day 7-

Breakfast
- fresh young coconut water (8 oz)
- pomegranate fruit (1/4 cup)
- raw hemp butter (2 tsp) on 1/4 gluten-free wrap or apple slices (1/4 apple)
- wheatgrass shot (1-2 oz)

Lunch
- fresh green and sprout salad with arugula, dandelion, sunflower seed and green pea sprouts (4 oz)
- grated avocado (1/3)
- black sesame seeds (2 tsp)
- balsamic vinegar (2 tsp)
- himalayan pink sea salt (optional)
- raw vegan zucchini and pistachio soup (3-4 oz)
- ginger shot (1-2 oz)

Dinner
- freshly made garlic hummus (3-4 oz)
- fresh cucumber slices & mini carrots (for the hummus - approx. 3-4 of each)

- side of fresh kimchi or sauerkraut (2 tsp)
- fresh parsley tea (1/4 bunch of fresh parsley boiled + simmered in water for 15-20 mms) - add natural sweetener if necessary (1/2 tsp)

Snacks
Avoid if possible. See pre- and post-detox sections for snack options.

16. HEALTHY MEAL PROGRAM (VEGETARIAN & NON-VEGETARIAN) - GUIDELINES

If you opted for the 7-day Healthy Meal Program, you can break the 7 days of detox into 1 day of pre-detox, 1 day of post-detox (using the specific guidelines provided in the appropriate sections of this manual) and follow the guidelines and recipes for the Healthy Meal Program for the remaining 5 days. Alternately, you may follow the plan for the entire 7-day period. You may also choose to extend the Healthy Meal Program for as long as you'd like after the 7-day period has ended, and eventually integrate the nutritious foods and super foods you used during your detox program into your daily food regimen for optimum daily detox, health and overall wellbeing.

Following are sample recipes you may want to use during your 7-day Healthy Meal Program. Alternately, you can hire a healthy cuisine chef or a local healthy meal delivery service if time is an issue for you and you have the budget for it. You may also use recipes from any healthy cookbook at your own discretion.

Remember that you can integrate any of the juices listed in the Juice Only Detox Program into your daily detox program if you wish to as long as your primary objective for detoxing is not weight-loss (since the addition of the juices will slightly increase your caloric intake. You can also choose to replace some of the healthy meals from your program with juices or smoothies. The combinations and options are endless. The only important rule to follow is that you consume your detox mixes, booster and juice/smoothie mixes daily, no matter how you decide to integrate them into your daily routine. See specific instructions under the appropriate sections that cover those detox supplements and detox instructions.

We classified meals by day for ease of reference. Feel free to rearrange your menu however you like and repeat meals that are particularly appealing to you as long as you vary the meals a little for fun, diversity and optimum nutrition. All ingredients in your meals should be organic and as fresh as possible into order to optimize detoxification and minimize further toxic exposure to your system.

Interestingly enough the emphasis is more about what not to eat rather than what to eat. Refer to the pre- and post-detox guidelines where we listed all the foods you should avoid during those critical times. This also applies during detox.

Day 1 -

Breakfast

- poached eggs (2 white, 1 yolk) or sugar-free muesli (1/2 cup) with sugar-free almond milk (1/2 cup)
- fresh (preferably unpasteurized) kefir (2-4 oz)
- fresh green or hot lemon tea - add natural sweetener if necessary (1/2 tsp)

Lunch

- tomatoes, cucumber, white onion salad w/ raw apple cider vinegar (RACV) & celtic sea salt

- tricolor quinoa with sliced avocado, steamed kale, fresh cilantro, gomashio (sea salt, sesame seeds and seaweed condiment)
- fresh dried herb thyme tea - add natural sweetener if necessary (1/2 tsp)

Dinner

- fresh carrot-ginger soup (4-6 oz)
- fresh tilapia steak or tempeh (4 oz)
- steamed spinach with fresh lemon, garlic and pink himalayan sea salt (4 oz)
- fresh parsley tea - add natural sweetener if necessary (1/2 tsp)

Day 2 -

Breakfast

- Bulgur hot cereal (1/3 cup), strawberry (2-3 sliced) and almond slices (2 tsp) w/ hemp milk (1/3 cup)
- fresh (preferably unpasteurized) kefir (2-4 oz)
- fresh green or hot lemon tea - add natural sweetener if necessary (1/2 tsp)

Lunch

- fresh mixed greens, sunflower sprouts, cilantro, fresh garlic, grated avocado (4-6 oz) w/ RACV & celtic sea salt
- black wild rice, lentils, onions, portobello mushrooms (4 oz), gomashio (sea salt, sesame seeds and seaweed condiment)

Dinner

- miso soup (6 oz) with shiitake mushrooms (4-5) and dried rehydratable Wakame seaweed (1 tsp)
- fresh brown rice sushi (mixed vegetarian or tuna rolls) (4-6 pieces)
- fresh edamame beans (organic only) (1/2 cup)

- fresh tulsi rose herb tea - add natural sweetener if necessary (1/2 tsp)

Day 3-

Breakfast

- fresh acai bowl (frozen acai berries, bananas) (4-6 oz), with optional fresh berries (1/4 cup) and a few banana slices (1/4) as topping
- fresh (preferably unpasteurized) kefir (2-4 oz)
- fresh green or hot lemon tea - add natural sweetener if necessary (1/2 tsp)

Lunch

- fresh lemon and garlic hummus ((4 oz) with fresh, uncooked broccoli, carrots, celery stalks (3-4 pieces of each)
- fresh baby greens, arugula, dandelion salad, cilantro, grated avocado (4-6 oz) w/ fresh lemon & celtic sea salt
- fresh herb peppermint tea - add natural sweetener if necessary (1/2 tsp)

Dinner

- fresh potato-leek soup (4 oz)
- brown rice, garbanzo beans, steamed veggies (4-6 oz), and gomashio (sea salt, sesame seeds and seaweed condiment)
- fresh herb chamomile tea - add natural sweetener to taste(1/2 tsp)

Day 4 -

Breakfast

- boiled eggs (1.5 white, 1/2 yolk) or breakfast polenta (1/3 cup), raspberries, blackberries, strawberries (1/3 cup), sugar-free

almond milk (1/3 cup)
- fresh (preferably unpasteurized) kefir (1-2 oz)
- fresh green or hot lemon tea - add natural sweetener (1/2 tsp)

Lunch

- fresh kale, pear, cranberries, sliced almonds, garlic, tahini, lemon and celtic sea salt (4-6 oz)
- oven-roasted root vegetable mix (yam, beets, butternut squash, parsnip, carrots, onions, thyme leaves, garlic, cannellini beans, hemp seeds, and celiac sea salt (4-6 oz)
- fresh fruit salad (berries, green apple) (1/3 cup)
- fresh ginger tea - add natural sweetener if necessary (1/2 tsp)

Dinner

- fresh and light gazpacho (1/2 cup)
- steamed Brussels sprouts, black quinoa, avocado (4-6 oz) (sea salt, sesame seeds and seaweed condiment)
- dark chocolate (85% or more) (1-2 small pieces)
- fresh parsley tea (drained water only) - add natural sweetener if necessary (1/2 tsp)

Day 5 -

Breakfast

- fresh green apple slices (1/3) with raw almond butter (2 tsp)
- fresh (preferably unpasteurized) kefir (2-4 oz)
- fresh green or hot lemon tea - add natural sweetener if necessary (1/2 tsp)

Lunch

- asparagus (4-6), pines nuts (1-2 tsp), lemon, tamari
- fresh flounder (4-6 oz), pepper, celtic sea salt, lemon or brown

rice and black beans (vegetarian) (4-6 oz)
- steamed green beans (2-4oz), garlic, sliced almonds, sesame seeds
- fresh ginger tea - add natural sweetener if necessary (1/2 tsp)

Dinner

- creamy mushroom and white bean stew (1/3 cup)
- steamed coconut infused rice (1/4 cup)
- fresh steamed vegetables, cashew nuts in coconut milk, spices(4 oz)
- fresh kava tea/drink - add natural sweetener if necessary (1/2 tsp)

Day 6 -

Breakfast

- fresh coconut with coconut flesh (1/4 flesh)
- blueberries and sliced banana (1/4 cup)
- fresh (preferably unpasteurized) kefir (2 oz)
- fresh green or hot lemon tea - add natural sweetener if necessary (1/2 tsp)

Lunch

- artichoke (1/4) , fresh garlic, lemon, and celtic sea salt
- gluten-free veggie wrap with carrots, beets, tomatoes, fresh hummus, avocado, cilantro, tahini, black sesame seeds, himalayan sea salt
- fresh ginger tea - add natural sweetener if necessary (1/2 tsp)

Dinner

- fresh herb salad (4 oz), grated avocado (1/4) , walnuts (2 tsp chopped), garlic, RACV, celtic sea salt
- fresh salmon (4 oz), sliced almonds, dill, parsley, minced scallions, lemon, pepper, celtic sea salt
- grilled vegetable brochettes (carrots, peppers, eggplant, sweet

potatoes, etc.) (4 oz)
- fresh mint leaves tea - add natural sweetener if necessary (1/2 tsp)

Day 7 -

Breakfast

- sliced avocado, blueberries, strawberries, bananas, raw almonds (1/2 cup)
- fresh (preferably unpasteurized) kefir (2 oz)
- fresh green or hot lemon tea - add natural sweetener (1/2 tsp)

Lunch

- tomato & portobello mushroom salad (4 oz) with fresh basil, lemon, RACV
- mashed sweet potato with coconut and lime (4 oz)
- lentils, carrots & onions soup (1/4 cup)

Dinner

- chicory salad (4 oz), pear (1/6), almond slices (2 tsp), dulse flakes, RACV
- freshwater trout (3-4 oz) with sliced raw almonds (2 tsp), fresh lemon, himalayan sea salt, pepper or tempeh (vegetarian) (4 oz)
- broiled yellow corn (1/2) and porcini mushroom (2-3)
- fresh ginger tea - add natural sweetener if necessary (1/2 tsp)

For specific recipes for all these meals, check online at www. thedetoxco.com.

17. ADDITIONAL JUICE RECIPES

To add a little more variety and versatility to your Juice Only Program, use the additional delicious detox juices listed in this section in addition (if you wish to increase your caloric intake) or as a replacement to the recipes listed in your Juice Detox program. You can also use these juices in Post-detox and thereafter, as part of your Daily Detox Maintenance Program in order to continue to benefit from daily detox and actively prevent excessive toxic exposure and build-up. Remember to choose organic ingredients only wherever possible. This is essential in order to support the safe and effective detoxification process during your program. Note that most of the juices listed below are much higher in sugar content (especially the ones that contain high sugar fruit) and should not be consumed if your primary objective for doing a detox program is weight-loss. If that is the case, stay with as many green juices as possible.

TOP DETOX JUICES

Simple Cleansing Green
- Green Apples* (4)
- Ginger (1/4 root - 2")**
- Lemon (1/2)

Sweet Digestion & Blood Cleanser
- Mango (1/2)
- Pineapple (1/8)
- Papaya (1/8)
- Fresh Aloe Leaf (1/8)
- Cucumber (1/2)
- Lemon (1/2)

Blood Purifier
- Mango (1/2)
- Cucumber (1/2)
- Green Apples* (2)
- Ginger (about 1/4 root - 2")**

- Lemon (1/2)

Sweet Body Detox
- Carrots (3)
- Green Apples* (1)
- Pear (1/2)
- Ginger (about 1/4 root - 2")**
- Lemon (1/2)

High Detox & Digestion Aid
- Lettuce (1/8)
- Cucumber (1/2)
- Tomato (1)
- Green Apples* (1)
- Lemon (1/2)

GREEN DETOX JUICES

Blood and Skin Cleanser
- Green Cabbage (1/8)
- Arugula (4 oz)
- Green Apples* (2)
- Cilantro (1/4 bunch)
- Lemon (1/2)

High Antioxidant Cleanser
- Cucumber (1/2)
- Brussels Sprouts (8)
- Green Apples* (2)
- Parsley (1/4 bunch)
- Lemon (1/2)

Colon Cleanser
- Green Cabbage (1/8)

- Mung Bean Sprouts (4 oz)
- Sunflower Seed Sprouts (4 oz)
- Green Apples* (2)
- Cilantro (1/4 bunch)
- Wheatgrass (add 1-2 oz shot)
- Lemon (1/2)

Full Body Cleanser
- Celery (3 stalks)
- Fennel (1/4)
- Green Apples* (2)
- Parsley (1/4 bunch)
- Lemon (1/2)

Skin Cleanser
- Celery (3 stalks)
- Cucumber (1/2)
- Green Bell Pepper (1)
- Green Apples* (1)
- Garlic (2 cloves +)
- Lemon (1/2)

SWEET DETOX JUICES

Sweet Slimming Green
- Pineapple (1/8)
- Cucumber (1/2)
- Spinach (4 oz)
- Fresh Coconut Water (6-8 oz)
- Basil (1/4 bunch)
- Lemon (1/2)

Immune System Booster
- Oranges (2)

- Grapefruit (1)
- Limes (1)
- Lemon (1/2)
- Cinnamon (2 tablespoons)

Sweet Cold Buster
- Carrots (3)
- Oranges (2)
- Ginger (about 1/4 root - 2")**
- Lemon (1/2)

Sweet Body Cleanser
- Carrots (2)
- Beet (1/2)
- Green Apples* (1)
- Cucumber (1/2)
- Ginger (about 1/4 root - 2")**
- Lemon (1/2)

Sweet Body Cooler
- Fresh Coconut Water (16 oz)
- Cilantro (1/4 bunch)
- Mint (1/4 bunch)
- Ginger (about 1/8 root - 1")**

* Green Apples preferred (if you have a sweet tooth, use Fuji apples as an alternative.)
** If you are a regular ginger user/ lover, you can add more ginger to taste.

18. ADDITIONAL SMOOTHIE RECIPES

To add a little more variety and versatility to your Liquid Only Program, use any of the delicious detox smoothies listed in this section in addition (if you wish to increase your caloric intake) or as a replacement to the recipes listed in your Liquid Detox program. You can also use these juices in Post-detox and thereafter, as part of your Daily Detox Maintenance Program in order to continue to benefit from daily detox and actively prevent excessive toxic exposure and build-up. Remember to choose organic ingredients only wherever possible. This is essential in order to support the safe and effective detoxification process during your program. Note that most of the smoothies listed below are much higher in sugar content (especially the ones that contain high sugar fruit) and should not be consumed if your primary objective for doing a detox program is weight-loss. If that is the case, stay with as many juices and low-sugar smoothies as possible.

Dr. Oz Green Drink
- Spinach (1cup)
- Cucumber (1/2 small)
- Celery (1 stalk)
- Parsley (1/2 bunch)
- Mint (1 bunch)
- Carrot (1)
- Apple (1)
- Orange (1/8)
- Lime (1/8)
- Lemon (1/8)
- Pineapple (1/8)

Energy Boosting Smoothie
- Almond Milk Yogurt (plain or coconut flavor) (4 oz)
- 100% pure Cocoa powder (1 tbsp)

- Creamy natural peanut butter (1 tbsp)
- Banana (1/2)
- Cinnamon (1/4 tsp)
- Ice cubes (4)

Vitamin C Smoothie
- Orange (1) (juice only)
- Cantaloupe (1/4)
- Strawberries (4 oz)
- Tomato (1/2)
- Ice cubes (4)

Vitamin Cocktail
- Papaya (1/8)
- Kale (4 oz)
- Spinach (4 oz)
- Banana (1/2)
- Green apple (1/2)
- Ice cubes (4)

Super Energy Smoothie
- Pineapple (1/8)
- Watermelon (1/8 small)
- Coconut water (6 oz)
- Baby spinach (4 oz)
- Blueberries (4 oz)
- Green apple (1/2)
- Banana (1/2)
- Ice cubes (4)

Paradise Smoothie
- Peach (1)
- Avocado (1/8)
- Strawberries (4 oz)

- Almond Yogurt (plain or coconut flavor) - 4 oz
- Pomegranate (1/8)
- Grapeseed oil (1 tsp)
- Pure vanilla extract (1 tsp)
- Ice cubes (4)

19. ADDITIONAL RAW VEGAN MEAL RECIPES

For additional recipes to use during your Raw Vegan Meal Program, please visit www.thedetoxco.com. You may also use the preferred foods (most detoxifying) listed below for inclusion in your daily meals before, during and after completing your detox.

For an example of what your daily menu could look like, use the following model;

AM
Fresh Green juice, or any other juice of your choice

MIDDAY
Fresh juice or smoothie, or fresh soup, or fresh salad

PM
(individually or any combination thereafter depending on your level of hunger)
- Fresh soup
- Fresh salad w/ seeds and avocado
- Small volume of whole grains (quinoa, brown rice, millet) (4 oz)
- Fresh wild or organic high-quality fish (4-6 oz)
- Fresh steamed or broiled vegetables (4 oz)

PREFERRED FOODS

VEGETABLES

- All dark leafy and cruciferous greens
* kale
* collard greens
* broccoli
* Swiss chard
* cauliflower
- dandelion
- artichoke
- asparagus
- leeks
- beet greens
- green beans
- spinach
- baby kale
- arugula
- romaine lettuce
- celery
- fennel
- cucumber
- all sprouts (sunflower, pea green, broccoli, alfalfa, mung beans, garbanzo beans, adzuki beans, black eyed peas, etc)

HERBS, ROOTS & SPICES
- Fresh cilantro
- Fresh parsley
- Fresh mint
- Fresh basil
- Curcumin (Turmeric)
- Cayenne pepper
- Thyme
- Fresh ginger
- Wheatgrass shot (daily where possible)

FRUIT

- Avocado
- Green apples
- All berries (acai berries, blueberries, raspberries, strawberries, Goji berries)
- Papaya (for digestion)
- Pineapple (small volume)

NUTS & SEEDS & ALL RAW BUTTERS (from nuts & seeds listed below)
- raw almonds
- raw walnuts
- raw pecans
- raw hazelnut
- raw pumpkin seeds
- raw sunflower seeds
- sesame seeds (especially black)
- hemp seeds
- chia seeds
- flax seeds (both whole and ground)

OILS
- Cold-pressed Extra Virgin Olive Oil
- Extra virgin Coconut Oil
- Sesame Oil (small volume)
- Raw Tahini (small volume)

GRAINS
- Sprouted Quinoa
- Sprouted Brown Rice

BEANS & LEGUMES
- Sprouted lentils
- Sprouted garbanzo beans
- Black beans

- Adzuki beans

FISH
(Only wild or organic farm-raised)
- Tuna
- Salmon
- Lean Meat Fish

(Check guidelines for frequency of consumption of all fish at - http://www.nrdc.org/health/effects/mercury/guide.asp)

BEVERAGES
- Alkaline water
- Bancha tea
- Fresh green tea
- Kombucha (non-alcoholic)
- Iodine water

SWEETENERS
- Raw Manuka honey
- Raw Agave syrup
- Blackstrap molasses

20. ADDITIONAL VEGETARIAN & NON-VEGETARIAN FOOD RECOMMENDATIONS AND POST-DETOX GUIDELINES

The following recommendations for foods to use during your detox, or before and after are based on the anti-estrogenic diet. This diet was developed by Dr Ori Hofmekler and is highly regarded by many doctors of both regular and alternative medicine as a powerful way to detox the liver, lose weight and keep it off, and to effectively remove overly estrogenic foods that tend to have a negative effect on our hormonal and overall body chemical balance from your diet, thereby limiting exposure and negative effects.

Here is some background on the Anti-Estrogenic diet and how it can help detox and heal your body. The main objective of an anti-estrogenic diet is to completely or substantially reduce estrogen levels in our bodies. Due to increasing pollution and excessive estrogen use and environmentally induced contamination through chemicals and hormones found in food, also called xeno-estrogens and phytoestrogens, or certain genetic conditions, high estrogen levels are causing chemical imbalances in our bodies (especially for men who are not supposed to have so much estrogen in their system.)

The anti-estrogenic diet seeks to lower estrogen levels by reducing foods with phyto-estrogenic content and endocrine disrupting effects. In addition, the diet promotes the consumption of food that contain chemicals that change the way estrogen is metabolized, such as the compound Indole-3-carbinol in cruciferous vegetables which may help in lowering excessive estrogen levels.

The reason why the anti-estrogenic diet is so effective is because of how it supports liver health and detox. The liver is the primary organ that breaks down estrogen, the hormone responsible for symptoms present in hormonal imbalances, PMS and menopause. Poor liver function results in excessive estrogen circulation in the system, leading to uncomfortable symptoms such as headaches, irritability, breast tenderness, pain with menstruation and mood changes. Constipation, or slow bowel transit time, tend to complicate matters further as the excess estrogen is not removed from the colon, leading to more estrogen being reabsorbed into the bloodstream. Many female issues, including uterine fibroids and ovarian cysts are estrogen-related, so is weight gain in both sexes. Therefore, decreasing sources of exogenous estrogen in the diet is highly advisable. Supporting optimal liver and bowel function is as essential since the liver is responsible for converting estrogen into an easily eliminated form supported by healthy bowels.

An anti-estrogenic diet has many benefits, including, but not limited to, improved libido and mental health, reduction of arthritis and cardiovascular diseases in men, reduced chance of metabolic syndrome, and long term weight-loss and weight management.

Following are general guidelines for the Anti-estrogenic diet, i.e. foods to avoid and those to consume frequently.

FOODS TO AVOID

The following foods should be avoided as they cause inflammation, smooth muscle contraction, vascular constriction, and promote inflammation and pain which in turn increases estrogen level and the production of more estrogen.

- Dairy (i.e. cheese, milk, cottage cheese)
- Methyl-xanthines -coffee, tea, chocolate, cola (minimize)
- Fat
  ✓ Animal fats - both meat and dairy
  ✓ Butter and margarine
  ✓ Meat and meat derived products
- White sugar, white flour and any other refined grains/flours

FOODS TO EAT

Consuming liver-friendly foods every day will help with reducing estrogen levels and increase detoxification effects. Those are best eaten raw, steamed, in a stir-fry (mostly water), or in soups or added to salads. Include (upon awakening), drinking half a squeezed lemon into lukewarm water (8-12 oz) to your daily regimen.

√ Alfalfa

√ Asparagus
√ Beets
√ Bok Choy
√ Broccoli
√ Brussels Sprouts
√ Cabbage
√ Carrots
√ Celery
√ Cauliflower
√ Collard Greens
√ Dandelion Greens
√ Dark Green Leafy Vegetables
  (endive, chard, spinach, etc.)
√ Fresh Green Peas
√ Kale
√ Artichoke
√ Lettuce
√ Okra
√ Potatoes
√ Rutabaga
√ Squash
√ Watercress
√ Yam
√ Lemon

OTHER RECOMMENDED FOODS

√ Legumes (dal) i.e. chickpeas, lentils, red beans, lima beans, pinto beans, mung
   beans, black beans, green beans
√ Rice - brown and wild rice – any variety except white rice
√ Fermented soy i.e. tofu, miso, aburage, atuage, koridofu, tempeh
√ Whole grains - such as millet, quinoa, kalmut, oats, buckwheat,
   etc. (favor non-wheat grains over gluten-rich ones)

✓ Probiotics- filled Raw Dairy and Kefir

RECOMMENDED SNACKS

✓ Fruit: apples
✓ Nuts: almonds, brazil nuts, chestnuts, hazelnuts, walnuts
✓ Seeds: flaxseeds, pumpkin seeds, sesame seeds, sunflower seeds
✓ Raw veggies: carrots, celery, broccoli, cauliflower, pepper
 (dip in fresh hummus, baba ganoush, bean dip, guacamole, etc.)
✓ Yogurt (plain organic, preferably unpasteurized)

RECOMMENDED MEAT

✓ Cold-water fish-salmon,
✓ Tuna
✓ Herring
✓ Artichokes
✓ Mackerel

RECOMMENDED SPICES & OILS
✓ All Indian spices
✓ Caraway
✓ Dill seeds
✓ Fennel
✓ Flaxseed oil (unheated)
✓ Garlic
✓ Ginger
✓ Honey or molasses
✓ Olive oil (unheated)
✓ Onions
✓ Parsley
✓ Turmeric

ANTI-ESTROGENIC DIET
Following are specific guidelines for a simple and highly
effective 2-week food-based detox program that you can follow

during your detox or add on after having completed your liquid or non-liquid detox. This is primarily targeted to liver detox and to lower excessive estrogen levels from the body. After the 2 weeks (sometimes up to 6 weeks, if you decide to lengthen Phase I & II to last 3 weeks each), you will go into Phase III, which encompasses the slow reintroduction of foods.

Phase I: Week 1 - Liver Detox

Objective - To cleanse and detox the liver, lower estrogen levels and burn fat. In this phase, the main source of fuel is carbs. It can be lengthened as desired to last for up to 3 weeks.

Foods to avoid -

- Processed Food including white flour and all refined grains
- Sugar (natural & artificial)
- Alcohol
- Coffee, Tea and Caffeinated Drinks
- Soft Drinks
- Regular Dairy (Cheese, Milk. Cottage Milk/ cheese)
- Chocolate
- Chemicals & Preservatives
- Trans & Partially Hydrogenated Fats
- Meat & Meat Products
- Butter & Margarine
- Any food that makes you feel tired or cause any reactive symptoms (observe, journal and listen to your body)
- Diabetics should stay away from grains, sugar and starchy vegetables

General Food Guidelines -

- Limit foods to mostly raw, anti-estrogenic fruits and vegetables

or their juices, and small servings of light protein such as raw yogurt, fertile organic eggs
- Under-eat in the morning and early afternoon hours through the consumption of light anti-estrogenic foods for optimum liver detox benefits
- Maximize liver detoxification with the consumption of non-estrogenic foods
- Use whey protein concentrates (esp. Warrior Whey) as a recovery meal for athletes and active individuals (20-30 g protein/ serving)
- Daily Fresh Squeezed Lemon in Hot Water upon waking
- If juicing, all juices should be made fresh
- Enjoy fresh Organic Green Apples & Ginger Juice daily
- Food should ideally be organic and fresh
- For smoothies, use a Vitamix, Healthmaster or Blendtec
- Use Spring Water/ Ice, Raw Milk (cow or goat), Almond or Hemp Milk as a base if making smoothies
- Use Anti-Estrogenic Spices & Herbs (as listed above)
- Focus on Soups, Salads, and favor Steaming & Broiling Foods
- If using oils/ fats, use cold pressed olive or coconut oil only
- Favor Manuka Honey or Molasses as a sweetener

Specific Foods to focus on -

- All Cruciferous Vegetables incl. Cabbage, Kale, Brussels Sprouts, Bokchoy, Cauliflower, Broccoli, Swiss Chard, Collard Greens and all Leafy Greens (Endive, Chard, Spinach, etc.)
- Green Vegetables & Others incl. Asparagus, Celery, Dandelion Greens, Lettuce, Okra, Fresh Green Peas, Artichokes, Watercress, Beets, Celery, Carrots, etc.
- All Sprouts (Alfalfa, Pea Greens, Broccoli Sprouts, Sunflower Sprouts)
- Favored beans: garbanzo, pinto and black beans, etc.,
- Favored grains: barley, oats, brown rice, quinoa, etc.

- Sesame Tahini, hummus
- Citrus Fruits (Lemon, Lime, Orange, Grapefruit)
- Omega 3 oils (hemp seed, raw flax seed - both ground & whole or unheated oil, sesame seed, E3Live, etc.)
- Organic Raw Dairy including aged cheese
- Best source of pesticide-free protein concentrate such as Warrior Whey Protein
- Organic Raw Low Fat Yogurt or/ and Kefir w/ Probiotics (active cultures) (up to 8oz)
- 1-2 fertile organic eggs (1 yolk only)
- Preferred Nuts & Seeds, all raw and organic, preferably rehydrated where possible - Almonds, Pecans, Walnuts, Pumpkin Seeds, Flax Seeds, Hemp Seeds and Chia Seeds
- Specific herbs and spices to integrate (All Indian spices, Caraway Dill seeds, Fennel, Garlic, Ginger, Onions, Parsley, Turmeric, Rosemary, Thyme, Oregano, Mandrake, Juniper, Mistletoe, Green Tea, Quercetin, Chrysin, etc.)
- Low Glycemic Fruit (esp. Berries and Green Apples)

Phase II: Week 2 - High Fat Diet

Objective - To promote anti-estrogenic hormones (progesterone for females and testosterone for males) and make Metabolism shift from Carb to Fat fuel. This phase can be lengthened as desired to last for up to 3 weeks.

Foods to avoid - (same as in Phase I.)

- Processed Food including white flour and all refined grains
- Sugar (natural & artificial)
- Alcohol
- Coffee, Tea and Caffeinated Drinks
- Soft Drinks
- Regular Dairy (Cheese, Milk. Cottage Milk/ cheese)

- Chocolate
- Chemicals & Preservatives
- Trans & Partially Hydrogenated Fats
- Meat & Meat Products
- Butter & Margarine
- Any food that makes you feel tired or cause any reactive symptoms (observe, journal and listen to your body)
- Diabetics should stay away from grains, starchy vegetables and sugar

General Food Guidelines - (similar to Phase I.)

- Under-eat in the morning and early afternoon hours through the consumption of light anti-estrogenic foods for optimum liver detox benefits, the main meal being the evening meal
- Incorporate the same Anti-Estrogenic foods as in Phase I
- Main source of protein now includes seafood (wild-caught)
- Increase consumption of Nuts and Seeds (use one at time to determine what works best for your body.)
- Best nuts to eat are almonds, pecans and walnuts
- Best seeds to eat are pumpkin, flaxseed, hemp seeds (freshly ground) and chia seeds
- Gradually incorporate one new food a day into the diet to see how the body reacts
- Focus on Sterol-rich foods such as Nuts, Seeds, Avocados, Olives, Stabilized Rice and Wheat Germ Oil
- Daily Fresh Squeezed Lemon in Hot Water upon waking
- Enjoy fresh Organic Green Apples & Ginger Juice daily
- Food should ideally be organic and fresh
- For smoothies, use a Vitamix, Healthmaster or Blendtec
- Use Spring Water/ Ice, Raw Milk (cow or goat), Almond or Hemp Milk as a base if consuming smoothies
- Use Anti-Estrogenic Spices & Herbs (as listed above)
- Focus on Soups, Salads, and favor Steaming & Broiling Foods
- If using oils/ fats, use cold pressed olive oil or coconut oil only

- Favor Manuka Honey or Molasses as a sweetener

Specific Foods to focus on -

- All Cruciferous Vegetables incl. Cabbage, Kale, Brussels Sprouts, Bokchoy, Cauliflower, Broccoli, Swiss Chard, Collard Greens and all Leafy Greens (Endive, Chard, Spinach, etc.)
- Green Vegetables & Others incl. Asparagus, Celery, Dandelion Greens, Lettuce, Okra, Fresh Green Peas, Artichokes, Watercress, Beets, Carrots Rutabaga, Squash, String Beans, Eggplants
- All Sprouts (Alfafa, Pea Greens, Broccoli Sprouts, Sunflower Sprouts)
- Citrus Fruits (Lemon, Lime, Orange, Grapefruit)
- Omega 3 oil (hemp seed, raw flax seed - both ground & whole or unheated oil, sesame seed, E3Live, etc.)
- Organic Raw Dairy (esp. Warrior Whey Protein)
- Organic Raw Yogurt and Kefir w/ Probiotics (active cultures)
- Organic Aged Cheese
- Preferred Nuts & Seeds, all raw and organic, preferably rehydrated where possible - Almonds, Pecans, Walnuts, Pistachios (optional), Pumpkin Seeds, Flaxseeds, Hemp Seeds and Chia Seeds.
- Sesame seeds or tahini (optional)
- Meat - Wild caught Cold Water fish-salmon, tuna, sardines, cod, orange roughy - preferably in non-polluted waters
- Seafood such as shrimp, lobster or crab
- Specific herbs and spices to integrate (All Indian spices, Caraway Dill seeds, Fennel, Garlic, Ginger, Onions, Parsley, Turmeric, Rosemary, Thyme, Oregano, Mandrake, Juniper, Mistletoe, Green Tea, Quercetin, Chrysin, etc.)
- Low Glycemic Fruit (esp. Berries and Green Apples) and Avocado
- Extra virgin, cold pressed olive oil

Phase III: Week 3 - Reintroduction of Foods

Objective - To promote anti-estrogenic hormones (progesterone for females and testosterone for males) and make Metabolism shift from Carb to Fit fuel. This phase can be lengthened as desired to last for up to 3 weeks.

Foods to consume sparsely - (same as in Phase I & II.)
- Processed Food including white flour and all refined grains
- Sugar (natural & artificial)
- Alcohol
- Coffee, Tea and Caffeinated Drinks
- Soft Drinks
- Regular Dairy (Cheese, Milk. Cottage Milk/ cheese)
- Chocolate
- Chemicals & Preservatives
- Trans & Partially Hydrogenated Fats
- Butter & Margarine
- Any food that makes you feel tired or causing any reactive symptoms (observe, journal and listen to your body)
- Diabetics should stay away from grains, starchy vegetables and sugar

General Food Guidelines -

- Reintroduce foods one at a time (in your evening meal) so that you may identify any food sensitivity and optimize your food regimen
- Observe and journal on how the body feels the next day
- Avoid all foods that make you feel tired or cause some sensitivity/ reactivity
- Watch out for gluten and remove it altogether from your diet where possible (wheat, rye, barley, oats, spelt, kamut). This is

a #1 culprit for allergic reactions/ sensitivities, especially in the U.S. where most wheat have been modified.

- Daily Fresh Squeezed Lemon in Hot Water upon waking
- Reintroduce Grass fed meats, organic raw dairy and whole grains if you ate them before.
- For optimum slimming and weight-loss, continue with the high-fat regimen, alternating days, and minimize your consumption of grains, starchy vegetables and higher glycemic fruits
- Keep 1-3 days of detox each week so that you may continue benefiting from liver detox and lower estrogen levels
- Cycle carb days (phase I) with high fat days (phase II)
- Do not mix carb-fuel foods with fat-fuel foods.
- Protein can be combined with both carbs and fats
- Limit your consumption of animal protein to 3 times a week (fish, seafood, and grass fed meats)
- Food should ideally be organic and fresh (fruits, vegetables and grains)
- Favor grass fed meats, wild organic fish and seafood, grass fed raw fertile eggs, organic raw dairy, etc.
- Avoid plastic containers, especially those that contain BPA, and metal cans for foods and drinks
- Avoid Estrogenic Herbs and other Products with high levels of Estrogen such as Licorice, Hops, Dong Quai, Black Cohosh, All Synthetic Hormones, Birth Control Pills, Soy, Red Clover, Verbana Mother Wort, and all Sunscreens that contain
- Use Anti-Estrogenic Spices & Herbs (as listed above)
- If you are diabetic or have high blood sugar levels, remove grains, fruits, sugars (Stevia, Luo Han, and Just Like Sugar are acceptable for diabetics) and starchy vegetables (such as potatoes) from your diet until your blood sugar stabilizes at less than 100 for a minimum of 6 weeks
- For an easily digestible source of protein, use Whey and most especially Warrior Whey
- If using oils/ fats, use cold pressed olive or coconut oil only

- Favor Manuka Honey or Molasses as a sweetener
- Continue with the foods you were focusing on in Phase I & II listed below

Specific Foods to incorporate in regular diet -

- All Cruciferous Vegetables incl. Cabbage, Kale, Brussels Sprouts, Bokchoy, Cauliflower, Broccoli, Swiss Chard, Collard Greens and all Leafy Greens (Endive, Chard, Spinach, etc.)
- Green Vegetables & Others incl. Asparagus, Celery, Dandelion Greens, Lettuce, Okra, Fresh Green Peas, Artichokes, Watercress, Beets, Carrots Rutabaga, String Beans, Eggplant, etc.
- All Sprouts (Alfafa, Pea Greens, Broccoli Sprouts, Sunflower Sprouts)
- Citrus Fruits (Lemon, Lime, Orange, Grapefruit)
- Omega 3 oil (hemp seed, raw flax seed - both ground & whole or unheated oil, sesame seed, E3Live, etc.)
- Organic Raw Dairy (esp. Warrior Whey Protein)
- Organic Raw Yogurt and Kefir w/ Probiotics (active cultures)
- Preferred Nuts & Seeds, all raw and organic, preferably rehydrated where possible - Almonds, Pecans, Walnuts, Pistachios (optional), Hazelnuts, Chestnuts, Pumpkin Seeds and Sunflower Seeds
- Meat - Cold Water fish-salmon, tuna, sardines, cod, orange roughy, herring, mackerel - preferably in non polluted waters
- Specific herbs and spices to integrate (All Indian spices, Caraway Dill seeds, Fennel, Garlic, Ginger, Onions, Parsley, Turmeric, Rosemary, Thyme, Oregano, Mandrake, Juniper, Mistletoe, Green Tea, Quercetin, Chrysin, etc.)
- Low Glycemic Fruit (esp. Berries and Green Apples) and Avocado

21. OPTIONAL DETOX YOGA PROGRAM

Pre-Detox

If you commonly experience constipation or sluggish bowel movement symptoms, practicing 'Legs-Up-The-Wall' right after consuming your early morning fresh squeezed lemon tea will help stimulate bowel movement. For detailed instructions on how to perform this pose, you can visit the following link at http://www.yogajournal.com/poses/690.

If you are interested in following a yoga program geared towards optimum detoxification before starting your detox, we encourage you to check out the detox yoga program specifically designed for daily detox and to support a full detox. Detox Yoga program at http://www.stepflix.com/#yoga/detox_yoga. Use promotional code ME23567 and get 1st month completely free.

Detox

If you continue to experience constipation symptoms after increasing your daily water intake to at least 8-10 glasses of water daily while doing your detox, keep drinking the fresh squeezed hot lemon tea and practicing 'Legs-Up-The-Wall' as recommended in the Pre-Detox sub-section above.

If you wish to start or continue to practice yoga in support of your detox program, use the detox yoga program specifically designed for daily detox and in support of full body, mind and heart detox. To access this Detox Yoga program, please visit http://www.stepflix.com/#yoga/detox_yoga. Use promotional code ME23567 and get your first month completely free. During the detox, we encourage you to practice the Nu-Detox Yoga class for optimum detox benefits.

Post-Detox

If you continue to experience constipation symptoms after completing your detox, keep drinking at least 8-10 glasses of alkaline water daily, as well as the fresh squeezed hot lemon tea and practicing 'Legs-Up-The-Wall' as recommended in the Pre-Detox and Detox sub-sections above.

If you wish to continue to practice yoga after completing your detox program in support of daily detoxification objectives and maintenance, use the detox yoga program specifically designed for daily detox and in support of full body, mind and heart detox. Detox Yoga program http://www.stepflix.com/#yoga/detox_yoga. Use promotional code ME23567 and get the 1st month free.

22. OPTIONAL EXERCISE PROGRAM (AS AN ALTERNATIVE TO THE DETOX YOGA PROGRAM)

If yoga is not your 'style', we still recommend that you exercise during your detox program in order to stimulate your lymphatic system, make you sweat and support the elimination of toxins and other waste material, whether organic or not, in the body. Sweating is very important in order to eliminate the toxins from the body, so is drinking so that you can move the toxins out of the body. So try to pick an exercise program that will make you sweat. If you are not physically fit enough yet, work slowly towards it and use spa treatment as an alternative to get the toxins out of your body (epson salt bath, detox algae body wraps, sauna, hammam, lymphatic drainage or deep tissue massage, castor oil packs applied directly to the organs to improve circulation and detoxification, etc. See section 25 below for more.) Exercise also improves mood, and helps reduce stress.

Preferred forms of exercise to replace detox yoga include; qi gong, tai chi, dance, swimming, low impact running, fast walking, tennis, boxing, other aerobic disciplines and Controlled Fatigue Training (CFT), a very effective technique to support optimum physical conditioning. Choose from any other sports that appeal to you. As long as you keep your body moving, that's all that matters.

Follow a program that elevates the heart rate to at least 60% of maximum for 30 minutes, five times a week.

23. OPTIONAL WELLNESS PROGRAM

In all 3 stages of pre-, post- and detox itself, we recommend that you add specific wellness treatments to prepare the body for detox, aid the process of detoxification and support the healthy removal of excessive toxins and waste material that are released in the body during detox. Here are a few suggestions well-suited body treatments. Include as many as you can and is enjoyable for you.

At Home
- Detox Baths (with the following formulation; epson salts (2 cups), baking soda (1 cup), essential oil of lavender drops) - x3/ day.
- At Home Self or Partner Massage (Foam Rollers, Hands & Feet, Whole Body, etc.) - x1/ day.
- Dry Brushing (with a dry brush starting from extremities working back towards the left side of the chest where main lymph node is located) followed with a cold shower and application/ massage using extra virgin coconut oil all over the body - x 2/ day
- Castor Oil Packs applied directly to the organs to improve circulation and detoxification (liver, gallbladder, stomach, pancreas, spleen, etc.) - x3/ day
- Honey Wraps (covering the entire body with honey and sitting with it on for at least 15 mns) - x1/ day
- All-Natural Enema system followed by a wheatgrass implant (only if you have experience with this type of treatment. If not, we recommend that you see a hydro colon therapist for safety and optimum results.) - x1/ day
- Ocean Bath (if you live next to the ocean) - x 1/ day

At The Spa
- Detox Algae body wraps
- Sauna followed by cold bath/ shower
- Hammam (wet sauna) followed by cold bath/ shower

- Massage (Lymphatic drainage, deep tissue massage, or anything else of your choice, etc.)
- Hydro Colon Therapy

24. OPTIONAL ADDITIONAL MINDFULNESS PROGRAM

The following mindfulness exercises are very simple and take very little time to practice and they can yield very powerful results to support your personal transformation and empowerment. You can do them all, or choose and pick what appeals most to you and feels like it would support your process the most. They can be done completely independently from anything else or as an addition to the detox yoga program which includes both breathing and meditation techniques.

- Clearly set your **Intention** for your detox
- Clearly define **Goals and Steps** that support the transformation you wish to achieve on the physical, mental and emotional levels of your being
- Use **10-Breath Meditation** every time you feel negative emotions rising up to the surface (simply taking 10 full slow, deep breaths and releasing the emotion you wish to dissolve)
- Use **Mantras** (if you already have a spiritual practice, or exploring the exciting world of mantras and positive vibrations that can help shift your reality)
- Use **Positive Affirmations** (good and simple examples include, 'I am beautiful', 'I am loved', 'I am bountiful', 'I accept myself fully', 'I forgive myself', 'I love myself', 'I understand myself', 'I care for myself', 'I matter', 'I am important', 'I deserve the best', and many more...)
- Make a **Gratitude List** that identifies all the people, events and things you are grateful for in your life and expressing gratitude for the good things to come (what you wish to manifest and experiencing what you feel when envisioning it.)

- Make a **Forgiveness List** of all the people and events that you may have interpreted as hurting you, or where you feel you have hurt them and have the genuine intention to forgive them and let go of any anger or resentment, be it towards yourself or them.
- Keep a **Journal** of your **Food** intake before, during and after the detox, noticing how certain foods affect your state of being and your emotions and also understanding what triggers you to eat and what your relationship to food is, most specifically the emotional component of it.)
- Keep a **Personal Journal** in all stages of the detox to express your feelings and emotions, both positive and negative and the conscious observation of your personal transformation. Use **Creative Writing** to release what needs to come out and emphasize and support what you wish to reinforce in life.
- Design your own **Detox Music playlist** that supports your mood and your desire to promote and sustain positive vibrations in yourself throughout the entire detox. If you are still in the process of developing energetic sensitivity, use existing **Inspirational Music** (classical, binaural beat technology, etc.) to help shift or simply support your mood when necessary.
- Use other **Breathing Techniques** (ujjayi breathing, left nostril breathing, yin wei breathing, etc...) to settle your mind and bring back harmony and balance when you feel stressed or unsettled (for specific techniques, check our YouTube Channel at www.thedetox.com/user/thedetoxco.)
- Use various **Deep relaxation and meditation techniques.**
- Use the Sedona Method (an extremely powerful release technique that transforms and releases negative feelings and emotions immediately.)
- Use the **Tapping Technique** (same as above.)
- Use anything else at your disposal that you know to be effective and transformational in the release of negative

feelings and emotions
- etc...

25. THANK YOU NOTE

As a closing note, I'd like to thank you for entrusting me with supporting your objectives of optimum physical, mental and emotional wellbeing. I am extremely grateful for the opportunity to be of service. When you detox, you make a serious commitment not only to detox on all levels of your being but also to use the detox benefits and the insights that you gained to propel you towards complete transformation. Learning to let go of what doesn't serve you and to only retain what is necessary to live a balanced and harmonious life gives you the opportunity to make new moment to moment choices and reach your highest potential in life.

26. DISCLAIMER

The information contained in this book is intended for educational and informational purposes only. The content does not replace advice, diagnosis or treatment made by a qualified medical professional. Always seek the advice of your physician or any other qualified health provider with any question you may have regarding a medical condition. Never disregard professional medical advice or delay in seeking it because of something you may have heard or read. The statements in this book have not been evaluated by the FDA or any medical professional and are not intended to diagnose, cure, treat or prevent disease. Every individual is responsible for the direction of his/her own personal health care.

www.ingramcontent.com/pod-product-compliance
Lightning Source LLC
Chambersburg PA
CBHW072249310526
45795CB00011B/574